# ICU Nursing Priorities for Stroke Patients

*Editor*

MARY P. AMATANGELO

# CRITICAL CARE NURSING CLINICS OF NORTH AMERICA

www.ccnursing.theclinics.com

*Consulting Editor*
CYNTHIA BAUTISTA

March 2020 • Volume 32 • Number 1

# ELSEVIER

1600 John F. Kennedy Boulevard • Suite 1800 • Philadelphia, Pennsylvania, 19103-2899

http://www.theclinics.com

CRITICAL CARE NURSING CLINICS OF NORTH AMERICA Volume 32, Number 1
March 2020 ISSN 0899-5885, ISBN-13: 978-0-323-71099-2

Editor: Kerry Holland
Developmental Editor: Laura Fisher

*Critical Care Nursing Clinics of North America* (ISSN 0899-5885) is published quarterly by Elsevier Inc., 360 Park Avenue South, New York, NY 10010-1710. Months of issue are March, June, September, and December. Business and Editorial Offices: 1600 John F. Kennedy Blvd., Suite 1800, Philadelphia, PA 19103-2899. Periodicals postage paid at New York, NY and additional mailing offices. Subscription prices are $160.00 per year for US individuals, $428.00 per year for US institutions, $100.00 per year for US students and residents, $206.00 per year for Canadian individuals, $538.00 per year for Canadian institutions, $230.00 per year for international individuals, $538.00 per year for international institutions, $115.00 per year for international students/residents and $100.00 per year for Canadian students/residents. To receive student/resident rate, orders must be accompanied by name of affiliated institution, data of term, and the *signature* of program/residency coordinator on institution letterhead. Orders will be billed at individual rate until proof of status is received. Foreign air speed delivery is included in all *Clinics* subscription prices. All prices are subject to change without notice. **POSTMASTER:** Send address changes to *Critical Care Nursing Clinics of North America*, Elsevier Health Sciences Division, Subscription Customer Service, 3251 Riverport Lane, Maryland Heights, MO 63043. **Customer Service: 1-800-654-2452 (US and Canada); 314-447-8871 (outside US and Canada). Fax: 314-447-8029. E-mail:** JournalsCustomerService-usa@elsevier.com **(for print support)** and JournalsOnlineSupport-usa@elsevier.com **(for online support).**

*Reprints.* For copies of 100 or more of articles in this publication, please contact the Commercial Reprints Department, Elsevier Inc., 360 Park Avenue South, New York, New York, 10010-1710; Tel.: 212-633-3874, Fax: 212-633-3820, and E-mail: reprints@elsevier.com.

*Critical Care Nursing Clinics of North America* is covered in *MEDLINE/PubMed (Index Medicus), International Nursing Index, Nursing Citation Index, Cumulative Index to Nursing and Allied Health Literature, and RNdex Top 100.*

# Contributors

## CONSULTING EDITOR

**CYNTHIA BAUTISTA, PhD, APRN, FNCS, FCNS**
Associate Professor, Egan School of Nursing and Health Studies, Fairfield University, Fairfield, Connecticut

## EDITOR

**MARY P. AMATANGELO, DNP, RN, ACNP-BC, CCRN, CNRN, SCRN, FAHA**
Nurse Practitioner, Neuroscience ICU for Neurology, Stroke and Neurocritical Care, Brigham and Women's Hospital, Boston, Massachusetts

## AUTHORS

**ANNE W. ALEXANDROV, PhD, RN, AGACNP-BC, CCRN, ANVP-BC, FAAN**
College of Nursing, The University of Tennessee Health Science Center, Memphis, Tennessee

**MARY P. AMATANGELO, DNP, RN, ACNP-BC, CCRN, CNRN, SCRN, FAHA**
Nurse Practitioner, Neuroscience ICU for Neurology, Stroke and Neurocritical Care, Brigham and Women's Hospital, Boston, Massachusetts

**CYNTHIA BAUTISTA, PhD, APRN, FNCS, FCNS**
Associate Professor, Egan School of Nursing and Health Studies, Fairfield University, Fairfield, Connecticut

**LINDA M. BRESETTE, DNP, MSN, NP-C**
Director, Comprehensive Stroke Program, Neurology, Brigham and Women's Hospital, Boston, Massachusetts

**WENDY DUSENBURY, DNP, RN, FNP-BC, AGACNP-BC, CNRN, ANVP-BC**
College of Nursing, The University of Tennessee Health Science Center, Memphis, Tennessee

**MARY McKENNA GUANCI, MSN, RN, CNRN, SCRN**
Clinical Nurse Specialist, Massachusetts General Hospital, Boston, Massachusetts

**KIFFON M. KEIGHER, MSN, ACNP-BC, RN**
Acute Care Nurse Practitioner, Neurosurgery and Neuroendovascular, Advocate Lutheran General Hospital, System Stroke Program Manager, Advocate Aurora Health, Chicago, Illinois

**MAUREEN LE DANSEUR, MSN, CNS, ACNS-BC, CRRN, CCM**
Sharp Memorial Rehabilitation Center, San Diego, California

**DEA MAHANES, DNP, RN, CCNS, FNCS**
Clinical Nurse Specialist, Neurocritical and Neuro Intermediate Care, University of Virginia Health System, Charlottesville, Virginia

**SARAH BETH THOMAS, MSN, RN, CCRN, SCRN, CNRN**
Professional Development Manager, Neuroscience/Critical Care, Brigham Health/Brigham and Women's Hospital, Boston, Massachusetts

# Contents

Acute stroke assessment is classically supported by clinical localization whereby presenting disabilities are associated with key arterial territories in the brain. Clinical localization skills are rarely taught to nonneurologists; yet, these skills are essential to the provision of evidence-based nursing care of stroke, enabling rapid patient identification, diagnosis, and ultimately, the delivery of acute treatment. This article explores the process of clinical localization in relation to the physiology affected by stroke vascular insufficiency. Elements of the neurologic examination are described as they relate to discreet areas in the brain and the National Institutes of Health Stroke Scale.

Acute ischemic stroke is a major cause of death and disability in the United States. Historically, acute stroke patients were treated with intravenous (IV) thrombolysis. Patients with large vessel occlusions (LVOs) should be offered mechanical thrombectomy, with or without IV thrombolysis, in an extended window up to 24 hours of last known well. Both treatment options are the standard of care for a patient with an LVO. It is critical that the intensive care unit nurse understand new treatment indications for LVO strokes, and the priorities of nursing care with medical and endovascular intervention.

Despite advances in understanding the cause of ischemic stroke, cryptogenic stroke remains a diagnostic and therapeutic challenge for clinicians. Approximately 15% to 40% of all ischemic strokes have no identifiable cause. CS is a diagnosis of exclusion after completing the standard stroke work-up. Further investigation needs to be tailored individually according to results of the clinical evaluation so appropriate secondary prevention strategies can be applied.

Malignant hemispheric stroke occurs in 10% of ischemic strokes and has one of the highest mortality and morbidity rates. This stroke, also known as malignant middle cerebral artery stroke, may cause ischemia to an entire hemisphere causing edema, herniation, and death. A collaborative interdisciplinary team approach is needed to manage these complex stroke patients. The nurse plays a vital role in bedside management and support of the patient and family through this complex course of care. This article discusses malignant middle cerebral artery stroke pathophysiology, techniques to predict patients at risk for herniation, collaborative care strategies, and nursing care.

Nearly 20% of all patients with ischemic stroke will require care in an intensive care unit (ICU), particularly those who have received intravenous alteplase or endovascular therapy. Prioritizing nursing intervention and intensive care monitoring can improve patient outcomes and reduce disability. A collaborative interdisciplinary team approach best facilitates the ICU care of an acute stroke patient.

It is unpredictable which stroke survivors will experience a seizure following a stroke. Stroke is a major cause of seizures. Critical care nurses need to know the risk factors, type of stroke at risk, stroke location, and severity for the poststroke patient who is at risk for an early or late seizure. Poststroke seizures require appropriate nursing assessments, management, and support.

Acute stroke care is completed, and it is time for discharge. Depending on patient needs, they may continue care with outpatient therapies, home health, long-term acute care, or an acute inpatient rehabilitation facility. This is an overview of the rehabilitation process, nursing care, an interdisciplinary team approach, and psychosocial aspects of acute inpatient rehabilitation. Rehabilitation nursing focuses on goals, outcomes, the attainment or maintenance of functional capacity, understanding long-range patient needs, and wellness. From the moment care delivery is initiated we should all be a part of the rehabilitation process, a link in the chain toward improved quality of life.

Many academic and community hospitals have obtained, or are considering obtaining, stroke center certification. Participation in structured quality improvement programs that also incorporate an objective assessment has been shown to improve outcomes and foster team building. Although obtaining certification can be challenging and costly, it can provide a framework to ensure hospitals deliver high- level, evidence-based stroke care. For the intensive care unit nurse, awareness and participation in the certification programs process is an important part of professional nursing practice.

Dea Mahanes

Stroke is a sudden, unexpected illness with an uncertain prognosis for functional recovery. Ethical issues in the care of patients with stroke include assessment of decision-making capacity when cognition or communication is impaired, prognostication, evaluation of quality of life, withdrawal or withholding of life-sustaining treatment, and how to optimize surrogate decision making. Skilled communication between clinicians and patients or their surrogates promotes shared decision making and may prevent ethical conflict. Nurses with an understanding of the ethics of stroke care play an important role in the care of patients with stroke and their families.

# CRITICAL CARE NURSING
# CLINICS OF NORTH AMERICA

---

**SERIES OF RELATED INTEREST**

Nursing Clinics of North America
http://www.nursing.theclinics.com

---

**THE CLINICS ARE AVAILABLE ONLINE!**
Access your subscription at:
www.theclinics.com

# Preface

# ICU Nursing Care of the Stroke Patient

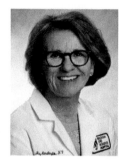

Mary P. Amatangelo, DNP, RN, ACNP-BC, CCRN, CNRN, SCRN, FAHA
*Editor*

Almost 25 years ago, in June 1996, the Food and Drug Administration (FDA) approved intravenous (IV) Alteplase as the only acute drug therapy for ischemic stroke. It remains the mainstay drug to date and revolutionized Neurology, Stroke, and Neurocritcal Care. In 2013, the success of several mechanical thrombectomy studies proved the efficacy of endovascular thrombectomy for large vessel occlusions (LVO), both alone and in combination with IV Alteplase. The expanded time window opened this treatment option to a greater number of patients, who are now surviving with fewer deficits.

The heterogeneity of the underlying disease process of stroke requires an interdisciplinary care team in concert to manage the complex stroke patient along the continuum. The constant in the process of stroke care is the bedside nurse. Fifteen percent to 20% of acute stroke patients will require management in an intensive care unit (ICU). The number of general ICUs far outweigh those that are neuroscience specific. Therefore, it is imperative for nurses working in the general ICU to be knowledgeable about caring for the stroke patient.

The aim of this issue is to review the major topics and controversies in caring for the complex stroke patient. Neuroscience nursing experts from across the country have been asked to contribute their expertise regarding key stroke issues. The goal of this issue was to provide a wide range of topics purposely selected to cover the continuum of care from localization, diagnostics, rehabilitation, and the ethical issues

Crit Care Nurs Clin N Am 32 (2020) ix–x
https://doi.org/10.1016/j.cnc.2019.12.001
0899-5885/20/© 2019 Published by Elsevier Inc.

ccnursing.theclinics.com

surrounding end-of-life care. It is our hope that this will contribute to improved stroke care and patient outcomes.

Mary P. Amatangelo, DNP, RN, ACNP-BC, CCRN, CNRN, SCRN, FAHA
Neuroscience ICU for Neurology, Stroke and Neurocritical Care
Brigham and Women's Hospital
15 Francis Street, BB 335
Boston, MA 02115, USA

*E-mail address:*
mamatangelo@bwh.harvard.edu

# Clinical Localization of Stroke

Wendy Dusenbury, DNP, RN, FNP-BC, AGACNP-BC, CNRN, ANVP-BC*,
Anne W. Alexandrov, PhD, RN, AGACNP-BC, CCRN, ANVP-BC

## KEYWORDS

- Acute stroke • Clinical localization • Arterial vascular territory • Stroke assessment
- National Institutes of Health Stroke Scale

## KEY POINTS

- Expert stroke nursing care is supported by knowledge of vascular anatomy in relation to brain parenchymal physiology.
- Clinical localization is the process by which stroke clinical findings are associated with affected arterial territories in the brain.
- Although clinical localization is rarely taught to nonneurologists, nurses caring for acute stroke patients must master aspects of the localization process to enable rapid diagnosis and treatment and facilitate evidence-based ongoing evaluation.

## INTRODUCTION

Clinical localization is the process of aligning stroke symptoms with specific vascular territories in the brain.[1–5] Although noncontrast computed tomography (CT) is essential to rule out hemorrhage, patients early into ischemic stroke (<6 hours) often present with normal CT scans; therefore, ischemic stroke is a clinical diagnosis dependent on localization of symptoms to specific arterial distributions. Localization is rarely taught to nonneurologists; it is a skill that requires knowledge of brain anatomy and physiology in relation to the arterial vasculature.[1,5] However, nurses intent on developing expertise in acute stroke are well served to understand at least the most classic stroke findings associated with arterial clinical localization to support their understanding of stroke progression or improvement, and to assist in prognostication of patient outcomes.

## CLINICAL LOCALIZATION OF ACUTE STROKE

The brain is made up of discreet sections that each have unique functions; when injured, these areas produce disabilities that examiners identify in symptom clusters

College of Nursing University of Tennessee Health Science Center, 920 Madison Avenue, Office Suite 568, Memphis, TN 38163
* Corresponding author.
*E-mail address:* wdusenb1@uthsc.edu

representative of discreet arterial brain regions. Localization is dependent on an understanding of the physiology within each area of the brain alongside the vasculature associated with these regions so that stroke arterial distribution is identified.[1,4]

### Brodmann Classification and Cortical Arterial Distribution

In the early 1900s, Brodmann[2] mapped what is called the "cytoarchitecture of the brain" (**Fig. 1**), a numbered system classifying cerebral cortical physiology in relation to autopsy findings demonstrating infarction or injury. Although the system is incomplete, Brodmann Classification remains the classic model informing practitioners today about discreet areas within the brain that are responsible for important cortical functions. Stroke clinical localization combines knowledge of Brodmann classification with an understanding of the vasculature that serves these regions, so that symptoms suggesting abnormal function may be associated with reduced blood flow in a discreet portion of an artery.[1]

The brain's arterial distribution is divided into anterior and posterior divisions (**Fig. 2**). The majority blood flow is directed to the anterior circulation of the brain, which is derived from the internal carotid arteries (ICA). In approximately 70% of individuals, the ICAs arise from the common carotid arteries (CCA) bilaterally, with the right CCA arising from the innominate artery and left CCA arising directly from the aortic arch. However, the most common arch variant occurring in about 13% of individuals is the "bovine aortic arch," where the left common carotid shares its origin with the right CCA in the innominate artery or it arises from the innominate artery more distally than the right CCA. Bovine aortic arch presentations are more common among blacks than whites, although the reason is unknown. Regardless of its origin, the CCA bifurcates into the external carotid artery, which goes on to supply the face and other

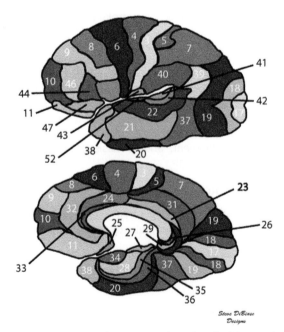

**Fig. 1.** Brodmann cytoarchitecture of the brain. (*Reprinted* with permission, Health Outcomes Institute, LLC, Fountain Hills, Arizona, USA.)

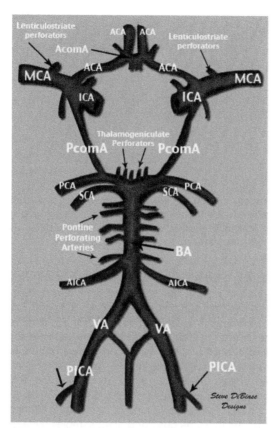

**Fig. 2.** Arterial vasculature of the brain. (*Reprinted* with permission, Health Outcomes Institute, LLC, Fountain Hills, Arizona, USA.)

head structures, and the ICAs, which travels deep within the brain, ultimately giving off the ophthalmic arteries (OA), the 2 posterior communicating arteries (PcomA), the anterior cerebral arteries (ACA), and the middle cerebral arteries (MCA). The posterior circulation of the brain is derived from the vertebral arteries (VA). The right VA arises from the innominate artery, which then goes on to become the right subclavian artery, and the left subclavian arises from the aortic arch and gives off the left VA. The VAs travel through the vertebral column winding their way up the neck into the skull, where they give off the posterior inferior cerebellar arteries (PICA) and the anterior spinal arteries. At the level of the pons, the VAs fuse to form the single basilar artery (BA), which ultimately gives off the anterior inferior cerebellar arteries (AICA), the superior cerebellar arteries (SCA), and at the most distal aspect of the BA, the posterior cerebral arteries (PCA). Both the anterior and the posterior circuits connect deep within the brain to form the circle of Willis.[3,4]

The 3 main pairs of arteries supplying the cerebral cortex are the MCAs (largest distribution covering the lateral and inferior aspects of the frontal, parietal and temporal lobes), the ACAs (covering the anterior and superior-medial aspects of the frontal lobes, and the superior-medial aspects of the parietal lobes), and the PCAs (covering the occipital lobe, lateral-posterior-inferior aspects of the parietal lobes, as well as the thalamus, and the superior aspects of the brainstem and cerebellum).[3] **Fig. 3**

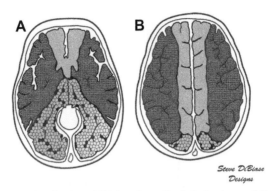

Fig. 3. Cortical arterial distribution. (*A*) View from the inferior base of the cortex. (*B*) Superior axial view of the cortex. Dark gray = MCA distribution; light gray = ACA distribution; speckled gray = PCA distribution. (*Reprinted* with permission, Health Outcomes Institute, LLC, Fountain Hills, Arizona, USA.)

illustrates cortical arterial distribution for the MCA, ACA, and PCA bilaterally; knowledge of this arterial layout is essential to support an understanding of cortical stroke clinical localization.[1] The first portions of the MCA, ACA, and PCA arteries before any bifurcation are commonly called the M1, A1, or P1 segments, respectively, whereas the segments after bifurcations are commonly referred to as M2, A2, or P2 segments; numbering of each of these divisions continues as the arterial distribution progresses further from their point of origin. The single anterior communicating artery (AcomA) is situated at the A1-A2 bifurcation connecting the right and left ACAs, whereas the 2 PcomAs, which originate from the ICAs bilaterally, move posterior, ultimately connecting at the P1-P2 bifurcation of the PCAs.[3] Although estimates vary depending on reports, as many as 50% of patient samples have been found to lack a "complete" circle of Willis; most commonly these anomalies involve one of the following[5]:

- A missing single A1 segment of the ACA with the remaining A1 segment supplying blood to the ipsilateral A2 segment as well as the contralateral A2 ACA segment via the AcomA;
- A missing P1 segment of the PCA with the PcomA supplying blood flow to the P2 PCA segment (referred to as "fetal origin of the PCA");
- A missing PcomA on 1 side.

### Relating Neurologic Findings to Arterial Distribution

A complete neurologic assessment is essential in all acute stroke patients. It must be performed quickly to collect assessment data and to assign specific suspect arterial territories in under a minute's time, to decide if findings do not follow a discreet territory, such as large intracranial hemorrhages that may cross arterial distributions, or to identify findings that are highly suspicious for a large number of stroke mimic diagnoses. **Table 1** presents findings aligned by vascular territories, anatomic structures, and assessment items on the National Institutes of Health Stroke Scale (NIHSS).

The NIHSS (**Table 2**) was originally developed for clinical trials of reperfusion therapies in acute ischemic stroke[6] and provides a structured method to tailor the neurologic assessment in a manner that allows practitioners to collect pertinent data and assign a score.[7–9] The NIHSS has a bias for left hemisphere MCA territory stroke in

**Table 1**
**Clinical Localization of Stroke**

| Lobe/Location | Function | Circulation | Neuro-vascular Territory | Common Pathologic Findings |
|---|---|---|---|---|
| | | | **Cerebral Cortex (Telencephalon)** | |
| Frontal Lobe | Voluntary motor function *Brodmann's Area:4* | Anterior | ACA (Superior-medial aspect) | • Leg Weakness *NIHSS Item: 6* |
| | | | MCA (lateral and inferior aspects) | • Facial weakness – *Central Cranial Nerve VII* *NIHSS Item: 4*<br>• Dysarthria (slurred speech) *NIHSS Item: 10*<br>• Dysphagia (difficulty swallowing) *Central IX & X Nerves*<br>• Arm weakness *NIHSS Item: 5* |
| | Broca's area *Brodmann's Area: 44*<br>• Expressive language (ability to name objects) | | MCA (usually left) | • Expressive Aphasia (inability to express language) *NIHSS Item: 9* |
| | Cognitive function *Brodmann's Areas:9–11*<br>• Orientation<br>• Memory<br>• Judgment<br>• Arithmetic<br>• Abstract Thinking | | ACA | • Orientation *NIHSS Item: 1B&1 C; influenced by NIHSS Item 9* |
| Parietal Lobe | Primary somesthetic sensory assessment *Brodmann's Areas: 1–3*<br>• Pinprick<br>• Vibration<br>• Position sense<br>• Temperature<br>• Touch | | ACA (Superior-medial aspect) | • Tactile Sensation (discrimination of pinprick) *NIHSS Item: 8* |
| | | | MCA (lateral and inferior aspects) | |

(continued on next page)

**Table 1**
*(continued)*

| Lobe/Location | Function | Circulation | Neuro-vascular Territory | Common Pathologic Findings |
|---|---|---|---|---|
|  | Somesthetic association of external stimuli spatial attention *Brodmann's Areas: 5,7* • Double simultaneous stimulation • Stereognosis • Graphesthesia |  | MCA (usually right) | • Neglect assessment (double simultaneous stimulation, tactile and visual) *NIHSS Item: 11* |
|  | Wernicke's Area *Brodmann's Areas: 37,39,40* • Receptive language |  | MCA (usually left) | • Receptive (Wernicke's or fluent) aphasia *NIHSS Item: 9* |
| Temporal lobe | Primary Auditory *Brodmann's Area: 41* |  | MCA | • Hearing loss; uncommon finding, generally not tested unless evident with sudden onset; central cranial nerve VIII *Not represented on NIHSS* |
| Occipital lobe | Primary Visual *Brodmann's Area: 17* Visual Association *Brodmann's Area: 18* | Posterior | PCA – Cortical vision MCA – Visual pathways OA – monocular blindness | • Vision; peripheral visual fields; differentiation between monocular and binocular lesions *NIHSS Item: 3* |
| **Subcortex** | | | | |
| Anterior, lateral and inferior white matter tracks | • Motor relay • Sensory relay | Anterior | ACA MCA Lenticulo-striate perforators | • Pure motor loss *NIHSS Items 4-6* • Pure sensory loss *NIHSS Item 8* • Mixed motor and sensory loss *NIHSS Items: 4-6 and 8* |

| | | | |
|---|---|---|---|
| Basal nuclei | | • Symmetric rhythmic movement<br>• Suppresses muscle tone<br>• Influences postural adjustments | • Pure motor deficit<br>*NIHSS: 5,6* |
| Posterior-lateral white matter tracks | Anterior | • Motor relay<br>• Sensory relay | MCA<br>Lenticulo-striate perforators |
| | Posterior | | PCA<br>Thalamo-geniculate perforators<br>BA |
| | | | • Pure motor loss<br>*NIHSS Items 4–6*<br>• Pure sensory loss<br>*NIHSS Item 8*<br>• Mixed motor and sensory loss<br>*NIHSS Items: 4–6 and 8* |
| Thalami | Posterior | • Relay of all sensory transmission except olfaction | PCA<br>Thalamo-geniculate perforators |
| | | | • Thalamic pain syndrome<br>*NIHSS Item 8*<br>• Pure sensory loss<br>*NIHSS Item 8* |

**Cerebellum**

| | | | |
|---|---|---|---|
| Neo-cerebellum (middle vermis, cerebellar hemisphere) | Posterior | • Projects fibers to the cerebral cortex through the thalamus; plays a role in planning and initiation of movements and regulating fine limb movement | BA<br>SCA<br>AICA |
| | | | • Ataxia and gait disturbances<br>*NIHSS Item: 7*<br>• Dysarthria (slurred speech)<br>*NIHSS Item: 10* |

*(continued on next page)*

**Table 1**
*(continued)*

| Lobe/Location | Function | Circulation | Neuro-vascular Territory | Common Pathologic Findings |
|---|---|---|---|---|
| Archi-cerebellum (Flocculo-nodular lobe) | • Processes impulses from the vestibular apparatus of the inner ear to maintain equilibrium, balance and posture <br> • Multiple connections with the ocular centers to facilitate eye movement in response to postural changes | Posterior | BA <br> AICA | • Vertigo, nystagmus <br> *Not represented on NIHSS* |
| Paleo-cerebellum (anterior lobe vermis, paramids, uvula, para-flocculus) | • Referred to as the spinocerebellum because it receives input primarily from the spinal cord; plays a role in control of muscle tone and axial limb movements | Posterior | PICA <br> BA <br> AICA | • Ataxia and gait disturbances <br> *NIHSS Item: 7* <br> • Dysarthria (slurred speech) <br> *NIHSS Item: 10* |
| **Brainstem** | | | | |
| Midbrain (Mesen-cephalon) | • Cell bodies for CN III & IV <br> ○ Pupillary constriction <br> ○ Eye movement <br> • Level of consciousness (ascending reticular formation) <br> • Ascending sensory tracts <br> • Descending motor tracts | Posterior | PCA <br> PcomA <br> Thalamo-geniculate perforators <br> Anterior and posterior choroidal arteries <br> SCA <br> BA | • Pupillary dilation <br> *Not represented on NIHSS* <br> • EOM dysfunction <br> *NIHSS Item: 2* <br> • Diplopia <br> *Not represented on NIHSS* <br> • Top of the basilar syndrome with cortical blindness <br> *NIHSS Item: 3* <br> • Decreased LOC <br> *NIHSS Item: 1* <br> • Motor/sensory pathway disruption <br> *NIHSS Items: 4,5,6,8* |

| Region | Structures/Functions | Circulation | Vessels | Clinical Findings |
|---|---|---|---|---|
| Pons (Meten-cephalon) | • Cell bodies for CN V-VIII<br>  ○ Facial sensation & jaw clench<br>  ○ Eye movement<br>  ○ Facial expression<br>  ○ Auditory reception & balance/equilibrium<br>• Pneumotaxic center<br>• Apneustic center<br>• Level of consciousness (ascending reticular formation)<br>• Ascending sensory tracts<br>• Descending motor tracts | Posterior | SCA<br>Pontine paramedian perforators<br>AICA<br>Internal auditory artery<br>BA | • Facial sensation<br>  *NIHSS Item: 8*<br>• Gaze palsies<br>  *NIHSS Item: 2*<br>• Diplopia<br>  *Not represented on NIHSS*<br>• Facial droop<br>  *NIHSS Item: 4*<br>  Note: *May present with bilateral symptoms, whereby the facial droop is ipsilateral to the pontine infarction and the limb weakness is contralateral to the infarction*<br>• Hearing loss; cranial nerve VIII; uncommon finding, generally not tested unless evident with sudden onset<br>  Not represented on NIHSS<br>• Decreased LOC<br>  *NIHSS Item: 1*<br>  ○ Locked-in syndrome<br>• Motor/sensory pathway disruption<br>  *NIHSS Items: 4,5,6,8*<br>• Respiratory arrest or insufficiency<br>  *Not represented on NIHSS* |
| Medulla Oblongata (Mylen-cephalon) | • Cell bodies of CN IX-XII<br>• Cardiac center<br>• Vasomotor center<br>• Respiratory center<br>• Level of consciousness (ascending reticular formation)<br>• Ascending sensory tracts<br>• Descending motor tracts | Posterior | PICA<br>VA<br>ASA | • Dysphagia<br>  *Not represented on NIHSS*<br>• Tongue deviation<br>  *Not represented on NIHSS*<br>• Decreased LOC<br>  *NIHSS Item: 1*<br>• Cardiopulmonary instability<br>  *Not represented on NIHSS*<br>• Vasomotor instability<br>  *Not represented on NIHSS*<br>• Sensory/motor pathway disruption<br>  *NIHSS Items: 4,5,6,8* |

**Table 2**
**National Institutes of Health Stroke Scale**

| | |
|---|---|
| 1a: LOC | 0 = Alert<br>1 = Arousable by mild stimulation<br>2 = Obtunded/arousable to pain<br>3 = Unresponsive/reflex only |
| 1b: Questions (month and age) | 0 = Answers both correctly<br>1 = Answers one correctly<br>2 = None are correct |
| 1c: Follows commands | 0 = Performs both correctly<br>1 = Performs one correctly<br>2 = Performs neither correctly |
| 2: Best gaze | 0 = Normal<br>1 = Partial deviation<br>2 = Forced deviation |
| 3: Visual fields | 0 = No visual loss<br>1 = Partial hemianopia<br>2 = Complete hemianopia<br>3 = Bliateral hemianopia/blind |
| 4: Facial palsy | 0 = Normal<br>1 = Minor<br>2 = Partial<br>3 = Complete |
| 5a: Motor left arm | 0 = No drift<br>1 = Drift<br>2 = Some effort against gravity<br>3 = No effort against gravity<br>4 = No movement |
| 5b: Motor right arm | 0 = No drift<br>1 = Drift<br>2 = Some effort against gravity<br>3 = No effort against gravity<br>4 = No movement |
| 6a: Motor left leg | 0 = No drift<br>1 = Drift<br>2 = Some effort against gravity<br>3 = No effort against gravity<br>4 = No movement |
| 6b: Motor right leg | 0 = No drift<br>1 = Drift<br>2 = Some effort against gravity<br>3 = No effort against gravity<br>4 = No movement |
| 7: Limb ataxia | 0 = Absent<br>1 = Present in 1 limb<br>2 = Present in 2 limbs<br>UN = Untestable |
| 8: Sensory | 0 = Normal<br>1 = Mild to moderate loss<br>2 = Severe to total loss<br>UN = Untestable |

*(continued on next page)*

| Table 2 (continued) | |
|---|---|
| 9: Best language | 0 = No aphasia |
| | 1 = Mild to moderate aphasia |
| | 2 = Severe aphasia |
| | 3 = Mute, global aphasia |
| 10: Dysarthria | 0 = No abnormality |
| | 1 = Mild to moderate |
| | 2 = Severe |
| | UN = Intubated or physical barrier |
| 11: Extinction/inattention (neglect) | 0 = No abnormality |
| | 1 = Extinction to 1 modality |
| | 2 = Extinction to >1 modality |

that 7 total points require intact language skills, so that left MCA stroke patients generally will have much higher NIHSS scores than patients with right MCA territory strokes of equal infarct size.[10] Despite this bias, the NIHSS is widely acknowledged to be the gold standard[6] for ischemic stroke patient assessment, and therefore, mastering use of this instrument is a prerequisite for acute stroke nurses.[11] Although the Glasgow Coma Scale (GCS) has been widely used as a neurologic assessment measure, the scale was originally developed as a level-of-consciousness (LOC) measure to prognosticate outcome in patients with traumatic brain injury.[12,13] In addition, GCS scores require recording the patient's "best response," so that in a stroke patient with normal LOC, the disabled side would not be scored if the tool were used correctly; in other words, despite being highly disabled, it is likely that a GCS may correctly score a patient as normal (score of 15).[13] Use of modified versions or what have been called "slim" versions of the NIHSS has been shown to be unacceptable by stroke nurses in that these scales may not capture the arterial territory affected by stroke, thereby giving false reassurance that a patient is not disabled when disability actually exists.[13] Therefore, the evidence-based recommendation widely accepted today is use of the full NIHSS, with use of just the NIHSS elements that are positive for the disability used during more frequent assessments for patients treated with alteplase (tissue plasminogen activator).[13,14] Recently, the NIHSS has been validated for use in patients with intraparenchymal hemorrhage.[15]

### Level of consciousness (National Institutes of Health Stroke Scale item 1)

Evaluation of LOC involves determining the degree of wakefulness in a patient and makes up one of the most important elements of the neurologic examination because it is a sensitive indicator of neurologic change.[16] Descriptors commonly used for LOC include alert (wide awake), lethargic (sleepy, dull, indifferent), obtunded (deep sleep; difficult to arouse), stupor (unarousable, yet with normal response [withdrawal or localization] to noxious stimuli), or comatose (unarousable with abnormal response [mass response or absent response] to stimuli).[17,18] Evaluation of LOC is included in NIHSS items 1a (wakefulness measure), 1b (responsiveness to questions), and 1c (responsiveness to commands). Generally, patients suffering anterior circulation ischemic stroke will have a normal LOC with the exception of catastrophic bilateral anterior circulation lesions[19]; this may remain true throughout the course of stroke completion with the exception of larger MCA stroke that is subject to severe or even malignant edema, which sets in and worsens within 24 to 28 hours after completed infarction.[20] Posterior circulation strokes are generally at greater risk of LOC deterioration, in particular, brainstem strokes, with disruption of ascending reticular formation and those affecting the cerebellum, which may cause brainstem compression and ventricular system obstruction.[1]

### Cranial nerve examination on the National Institutes of Health Stroke Scale

There are 12 pairs of cranial nerves (CN) that are generally classified as part of the peripheral nervous system; however, this is anatomically inaccurate in that CN II originates anatomically from the central nervous system.[4] A detailed description of CN anatomy and assessment is an article in and of itself, but suffice it to say that CNs I and III–XII are considered true peripheral nerves, whereas CN II (optic nerve) is derived from the optic stalks of the diencephalon composed of retinal ganglion cell axons and glial cells, and similar to other axons of the central nervous system, covered with myelin. Assessment of CN I (olfactory), which originates in the forebrain, is generally deferred, whereas assessments of CNs III–VII, which have their cell bodies in the brainstem, are incorporated within the NIHSS (see **Table 1**) with the exception of pupillary constriction to light, which can be added in the case of altered LOC or findings consistent with palsies of CNs affecting extraocular movement (EOM; CNs III, IV, and VI).[1,4] CNs IX, X, and XII make up important components of stroke patient assessment in that swallow integrity is insulted in about 50% of stroke patients[21,22]; swallow assessment will not be discussed in this article but often involves a comprehensive battery of tests starting with a clinical bedside screen, assessment of LOC which must be assessed to ensure adequate intake and airway protection, and fiber-optic endoscopic evaluation of swallow completed by a speech and language pathologist.[23] In addition, insults to CNs VII, IX, and/or XII may also impact speech articulation, resulting in a dysarthric quality that may significantly limit communication. Assessment of CN XI (spinal accessory) can be easily incorporated into a neurologic examination through the addition of shoulder shrug and head turning.[24] CN VIII (vestibulocochlear) is rarely tested unless the patient presents with stroke symptoms accompanied by a sudden-onset acute hearing loss or acute onset of vertigo; when this is the case, suspicion for brainstem infarction should remain high, especially when accompanied by other brainstem findings, although temporal lobe infarction may be a consideration.[25]

### Extraocular movement (National Institutes of Health Stroke Scale item 2)

Assessment of extraocular movements (EOM) provides the examiner with information reflective of brainstem integrity and level of brainstem dysfunction given that the cell bodies of these nerves originate in the midbrain (CN III and IV) and pons (CN VI).[26] Classically, the patient is asked to move his or her eyes to trace the movement of the examiner's fingers, generally in an "H" configuration, whereas the NIHSS asks the patient to trace the examiner's fingers through lateral eye movement.[19] In the case of altered LOC, oculocephalic maneuver or doll's eyes are examined, and an absence of full movement would indicate brainstem dysfunction.[27] In the conscious patient who is unable to understand what the examiner requests, the examiner should move about the patient to draw eye movement in his or her direction so EOMs can be evaluated.[19]

Findings from EOM testing must be differentiated from findings associated with the frontal eye fields (see **Fig. 1**; between Brodmann areas 4, 6, and 8, by the middle frontal and precentral gyri). The frontal eye fields are responsible for saccadic eye movements that normally allow the eyes to rapidly move together to surveil visual content; interruption of this area of the brain causes conjugate eye deviation toward the affected MCA territory.[28] In contrast, brainstem CN III, IV, and VI findings would include either lateral deviation, ptosis, and pupillary dilation (CN III;

oculomotor), loss of superior oblique innervation with upward migration and vertical diplopia that worsens when attempting to look down (CN IV; trochlear), or midline eye deviation with limited lateral gaze producing diplopia (CN VI; abducens).[27] With significant brainstem destruction, patients may present with a fixed gaze in combination with other classic brainstem findings, such as decreased LOC, including coma.[29]

### Peripheral vision (National Institutes of Health Stroke Scale item 3)

Peripheral vision (CN II) is assessed by evaluating each eye independently and both eyes collectively.[19] Vision for each eye is divided into 4 quadrants, and visual loss is determined to be either monocular (resulting from prechiasmal stroke affecting the retina or optic nerves) or binocular (stroke at or posterior to the chiasm).[1,19] The more posterior along the visual tracts that the stroke occurs, the more congruent the deficit is in each eye.[1,30] Visual field loss can be affected by the OA (monocular), MCA (binocular), PCA (binocular), or top of the BA (binocular, including bilateral hemianopia, also referred to as cortical blindness) stroke.[29] In the case of MCA stroke producing visual loss, the examiner should expect vision loss to also be accompanied by findings classically associated with MCA stroke, such as voluntary motor and/or primary sensory loss, aphasia (usually left hemisphere), and/or neglect (usually right hemisphere),[29,31] whereas in pure P2 PCA stroke, the examiner would expect binocular hemianopia without other disability findings.[32]

To evaluate visual fields, the examiner assesses the patient's ability to visualize an object (usually the examiner's fingers) in each of the 4 quadrants of vision.[19] Although some NIHSS training films demonstrate this assessment by asking the patient to state how many fingers he or she is able to see in each field, this often leads to confusion. For example, if the patient says "2 fingers" when 3 fingers were actually held up, some examiners miss-score this as visual field loss; however, the patient did in fact see the examiner's fingers, so vision should be assumed to be intact. The error in this example may actually be on the part of the examiner through failure to accurately position fingers within the patient's visual field. Therefore, it is often clearer to just simply have the patient state "now" when he or she sees the examiner's finger start wiggling in each quadrant. However, by far the most common error made by novice examiners is holding their arms/fingers too far into the periphery for the patient to see. Examiners must remember to use themselves as confirmation and make sure that their fingers are held well within a field of vision that is easily seen to avoid assuming visual loss in a patient who has normal visual fields. For patients unable to participate in this examination because of altered LOC, cognitive or language dysfunction, blinking-to-threat will suffice as confirmation of intact vision.[28]

### Facial symmetry (National Institutes of Health Stroke Scale item 4)

Nervous control of facial expression arises from the corticobulbar fibers that originate on the lower lateral side of the precentral gyrus (see **Fig. 1**; Brodmann area 4; MCA territory), coursing through the corona radiata, internal capsule, and medial cerebral peduncle to the pons where most fibers decussate and then terminate in the contralateral facial motor cell body.[1] Stroke affecting the MCA territory interferes with precentral gyrus transmission, producing what is often referred to as "central VII" motor loss, whereas brainstem stroke at the site of the pontine CN VII nucleus results in loss of peripheral facial innervation. With central VII loss, the upper face is commonly spared, and there are several physiologic theories explaining this preserved function, including bilateral supranuclear control and the scant direct cortical innervation provided to the upper face. Therefore, loss of the upper face is expected to occur most commonly with brainstem pontine stroke and is considered uncommon in MCA distribution stroke.[1,33] Assessment of symmetric facial expression (CN VII) is assessed by asking the patient to smile, blow out the cheeks, close the eyes tightly, and raise the eyebrows.[19] Dysarthria or slurred speech (NIHSS item 10) is commonly found in relation to motor loss affecting the lower face.[19] Expected findings align with vascular territories as follows:

- MCA stroke: flattening of the nasolabial folds on the same side as limb weakness[1]
- BA distribution stroke:[1]
  - Upper brainstem, coextensive (face, arm, leg) contralateral weakness in relation to the infarction
  - Lower pontine, facial droop ipsilateral to the pontine infarction with limb weakness contralateral to pontine infarction.

With extremely rare exceptions caused by discreet medullary stroke lesions (Dejerine anterior bulbar[1,34] [medial medullary] syndrome or pure Wallenberg [lateral medullary] syndrome that excludes Opalski[35] [submedullary] components), examiners should be highly suspect of presentations involving motor loss of the limbs with sparing of the face because this presentation may suggest a stroke mimic diagnosis. Completion of emergent MRI, diffusion-weighted imaging/apparent diffusion coefficient, and fluid attenuated inversion recovery sequences will immediately confirm or dispel stroke diagnosis with such a presentation.[36]

### Motor Examination on the National Institutes of Health Stroke Scale

The motor homunculus, Latin for "little man" (**Fig. 4**), is a graphic depiction of what a man would look like if the body parts were proportionate to the amount/size of brain territory on the precentral gyrus (see **Fig. 1**; Brodmann area 4) dedicated to specific types of motor function. The most superior and medial areas of the precentral gyrus

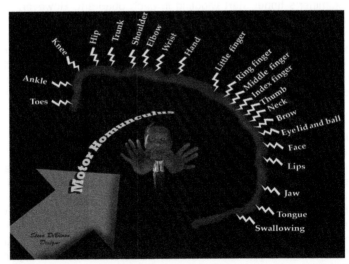

**Fig. 4.** Motor homunculus. (*Reprinted* with permission, Health Outcomes Institute, LLC, Fountain Hills, Arizona, USA.)

control voluntary movement for the lower extremities; progressing laterally and inferiorly, the homunculus distribution includes the trunk, arm, hand, face, lips, tongue, and larynx. When considering the layout of the motor homunculus in relation to the anterior circulation's distribution, the ACA supplies blood flow to the areas of the precentral gyrus that innervate voluntary motor function in the lower limbs, whereas MCA distribution supplies blood flow to areas on the gyrus responsible for innervation of the arms and facial and orolingual structures. For this reason, MCA distribution strokes commonly present with similar motor loss in the face and arm; the more distal the MCA occlusion, leg involvement may be entirely spared, whereas in distal ICA/proximal MCA stroke near in proximity to the ACA A1 division (see **Fig. 2**), patients may present with face, arm, and leg motor loss.[1]

A large portion of the corticospinal tract originates in the precentral gyrus and descends through the internal capsule into the brainstem where most motor fibers decussate in the pyramids of the medulla before descending to the spinal cord and lower motor neurons. In this way, the right and left precentral gyri control voluntary motor function for the opposite sides of the body. Stroke that interferes with the descent and distribution of the corticospinal tract within the cortex, subcortex, or brainstem will cause voluntary limb motor loss on the opposite side of the body; Opalski syndrome complicating a Wallenberg presentation is a rare exception in that motor extremity loss is ipsilateral to the medullary stroke.[1]

Motor function is classically graded using a muscle strength scale of 0 to 5, where 0 equals no movement and 5 equals normal power (**Box 1**)[1]; findings are presented as a fraction with the patient's actual muscle strength in the numerator and normal muscle strength (grade 5) in the denominator. Motor function is also measured on the NIHSS in item 5 (motor arm) and item 6 (motor leg)[19,37]; the number assigned on the NIHSS should not be confused with the motor grade in that the NIHSS is a scale of which numeric values add weight to connotative severity on an ordinal scale.

Ataxia is a disturbance of smooth performance of voluntary motor function, resulting in errors in movement timing, force, range, and speed.[38] Stroke affecting the cerebellum results in motor function without inhibition and modulation, producing inaccurate and inconsistent movement.[39] Ataxia is tested on the NIHSS (item 7) using the finger-nose-finger, and heel-shin tests. The examiner has the patient reach using the full length of his or her arm to touch the examiner's finger; the examiner can move placement of his or her finger with each subsequent reach by the patient, while observing for smooth, accurate movement. The heel-shin test is performed with the patient lying on his or her back. The patient is asked to run his or her heel down the shin of the opposite leg and back up again to the knee; the test is repeated in both limbs while the examiner observes for smooth, accurate limb motion.[19] Misinterpretation of ataxia findings is common. When

---

**Box 1**
**Muscle strength grading**

0 = No muscle activation

1 = Trace muscle activation, such as a twitch, without achieving full range of motion

2 = Muscle activation with gravity eliminated, achieving full range of motion

3 = Muscle activation against gravity, full range of motion

4 = Muscle activation against some resistance, full range of motion

5 = Muscle activation against the examiner's full resistance, full range of motion .

motor weakness results in loss of coordination, ataxia should be scored as a 0 on the NIHSS; however, when motor strength is normal, but movement lacks coordination, ataxia should be scored as present.[19]

### Sensory Examination

Sensory pathways ascend the spinal cord decussating within either the cord or the brainstem before reaching the thalamus where they are relayed to the parietal lobe's postcentral gyrus.[1] The postcentral gyrus (see **Fig. 1**; Brodmann areas 1–3) houses the primary somatosensory cortex and can be illustrated with a sensory homunculus of which the layout is distributed by the amount of gyrus brain tissue dedicated to various parts of the body.[1]

Proprioception has a conscious and an unconscious component. The conscious pathway connects with the thalamus and the cerebral cortex, enabling an understanding of the position of the body in space, whereas the unconscious pathway connects with the cerebellum, facilitating walking and complex acts without having to think about which joints to flex and or extend. Although proprioception is not included as part of the NIHSS, it can be easily added to the neurologic examination when other sensory findings are identified; the test is performed with the patient's eyes closed, and the examiner then moves the patient's finger up or down, right or left, asking the patient what direction the joint is moving in.[1,40]

Examination of primary sensory function on the NIHSS includes testing of touch sensation on the face, arms, and legs. The examiner begins by touching the side that appears unaffected by stroke with a pin and asking the patient if it feels "sharp"; the examiner then moves to the affected side, repeating the procedure and asking the patient if it feels "as sharp" as the unaffected side. It is important to use a pin so that the patient can clearly discriminate the sensation, because use of touch alone may mask an actual sensory loss.[19]

In general, the right hemisphere dominates in completion of tasks that require nonvisual spatial attention, especially in right-handed persons.[41–43] Attention activated by external stimuli is localized to the inferior parietal lobe and the posterior aspect of the superior temporal gyrus with the right hemisphere alerting both sides of the body[1]; because of this, hemineglect syndromes are most commonly associated with right parietal MCA lesions.[44]

The NIHSS assessment of neglect (item 11) includes a tactile and a visuospatial component. Tactile neglect is tested with the patient's eyes closed to determine if the patient can distinguish being touched simultaneously on each side; in the case of left hemineglect syndrome, the patient is unable to consistently recognize simultaneous touch on the left side of his or her body. The examiner touches 1 side of the face or both sides of the face simultaneously with a brief on-off low-pressure movement and asks the patient to state which side was touched; the procedure is then repeated in the patient's arms and, if necessary, legs.[19] Visuospatial neglect is tested during assessment of NIHSS item 3 (to avoid redundant eye testing) in patients with intact visual fields, and findings are incorporated into the scoring of neglect on item 11. The examiner positions his or her fingers within the visual fields of both the patient's eyes; most commonly, the examiner asks the patient to state which finger is wiggling, right, left, or both, starting first by wiggling a finger on 1 hand, then the other hand, and then providing double simultaneous stimuli by wiggling a finger on both hands at the same time. Patients with hemineglect may present with only tactile or visuospatial neglect, or they may present with profound neglect, whereby both tactile and visuospatial attention are affected.[1,19,45]

### Language

Language is considered a sensorimotor function of the brain in that it requires functions tied to receiving and processing language (sensory) as well as language expression (motor).[1] In general, the left hemisphere of the brain houses language and linguistic functions, along with other executive functions, such as mathematical skills, reasoning, and analysis.[1] Aphasia is the inability to comprehend or formulate language[46] and is tested by NIHSS item 9.[19] Motor language aphasia produces expressive loss because of frontal cortical MCA stroke in the Broca area[47] (see **Fig. 1**; Brodmann area 44) and is tested through examination of language fluency on the NIHSS by asking the patient to name items and describe a scene.[19,48] Sensory language aphasia produces an inability to receive language because of MCA stroke in Wernicke area (see **Fig. 1**; Brodmann area 37, 39, and 40), resulting in an inability to assemble phonemes accurately, an inability to repeat sentences correctly, and an inability to name items correctly.[19,49,50] However, compared with those with Broca aphasia, patients with Wernicke aphasia have effortless, yet difficult-to-decipher speech, and therefore, this type of disability is often described as a "fluent aphasia."[51] The NIHSS item 9 assesses receptive deficits by examining language fluency as the patient describes pictures and reads sentences; the examiner can also attempt to engage the patient in conversation to further differentiate aphasia type.[19] Global aphasia presentations are associated with large left MCA stroke, often presenting with perisylvian lesions, that produce both Wernicke and Broca aphasia components, leaving the patient mute with impaired comprehension.[46]

## SUMMARY

A thorough and precise neurologic examination is essential to rapid diagnosis, treatment, and ongoing evaluation of acute stroke patients. Although challenging, practice and repetition, alongside a commitment to furthering knowledge of neurologic anatomy and physiology, are the keys to examiner proficiency and expertise. Subtle neurologic changes requiring immediate intervention often can only be identified through completion of serial assessments. Because stroke evolves over minutes to even days, nurses caring for acute stroke patients must seek to master assessment skills with an eye to the vascular territory affected to reduce significant risks for devastating disability, deterioration, and death.

## DISCLOSURE

The authors have nothing to disclose.

## REFERENCES

1. Brazis P, Masdeu JC, Biller J. Localization in clinical neurology. Philadelphia: Lippincott Williams & Wilkins; 2016.
2. Brodmann K. Vergleichende Lokalisationslehre der Großhirnrinde. Leipzig (Germany): Barth; 1909.
3. Chandra A, Li WA, Stone CR, et al. The cerebral circulation and cerebrovascular disease I: anatomy. Brain Circ 2017;3(2):45–56.
4. Alexandrov AW. Association of neurovascular clinicians core curriculum for neurovascular nursing. Fountain Hill (AZ): Health Outcomes Institute, Inc; 2012.
5. Iqbal S. A comprehensive study of the anatomical variations of the circle of Willis in adult human brains. J Clin Diagn Res 2013;7(11):2423–7.

6. Lyden P. Using the National Institutes of Health Stroke Scale: a cautionary tale. Stroke 2017;48(2):513–9.

7. Brott TG, Adams HP, Olinger CP, et al. Measurements of acute cerebral infarction: a clinical examination scale. Stroke 1989;20(7):864–70.

8. Brott T, Marler JR, Olinger CP, et al. Measurements of acute cerebral infarction: lesion size by computed tomography. Stroke 1989;20(7):871–5.

9. Lyden P, Brott T, Tilley B, et al. Improved reliability of the NIH Stroke Scale using video training. NINDS TPA Stroke Study Group. Stroke. 1994;25(11):2220–6.

10. Woo D, Broderick JP, Kothari RU, et al. Does the National Institutes of Health Stroke Scale favor left hemisphere strokes? NINDS t-PA Stroke Study Group. Stroke 1999;30(11):2355–9.

11. Goldstein LB, Samsa GP. Reliability of the National Institutes of Health Stroke Scale. Extension to non-neurologists in the context of a clinical trial. Stroke 1997;28(2):307–10.

12. Teasdale G, Jennett B. Assessment of coma and impaired consciousness. A practical scale. Lancet 1974;2(7872):81–4.

13. Nye BR, Hyde CE, Tsivgoulis G, et al. Slim stroke scales for assessing patients with acute stroke: ease of use or loss of valuable assessment data? Am J Crit Care 2012;21(6):442–8.

14. Middleton S, Grimley R, Alexandrov AW. Triage, treatment, and transfer: evidence-based clinical practice recommendations and models of nursing care for the first 72 hours of admission to hospital for acute stroke. Stroke 2015;46(2):e18–25.

15. Dusenbury W, Tsivgoulis G, Brewer Barbara B, et al. Abstract WP456: validation of the NIH Stroke Scale Score for clinical assessment of intracerebral hemorrhage. Stroke 2019;50(Suppl 1).

16. Dávalos A, Toni D, Iweins F, et al. Neurological deterioration in acute ischemic stroke: potential predictors and associated factors in the European Cooperative Acute Stroke Study (ECASS) I. Stroke 1999;30(12):2631–6.

17. Tindall SC. Level of consciousness. In: Walker HK, Hall WD, Hurst JW, editors. Clinical methods: the history, physical, and laboratory examinations. 3rd edition. Boston: Butterworths; 1990. Available at: http://www.ncbi.nlm.nih.gov/books/NBK380/. Accessed July 30, 2019.

18. Fisher CM. The neurological examination of the comatose patient. Acta Neurol Scand 1969;45(S36):5–56.

19. NINDS Know Stroke Campaign–NIH stroke scale. Available at: https://www.stroke.nih.gov/resources/scale.htm. Accessed July 30, 2019.

20. Hacke W, Schwab S, Horn M, et al. "Malignant" middle cerebral artery territory infarction: clinical course and prognostic signs. Arch Neurol 1996;53(4):309–15.

21. Martino R, Foley N, Bhogal S, et al. Dysphagia after stroke. Stroke 2005;36(12):2756–63.

22. Aviv JE, Martin JH, Sacco RL, et al. Supraglottic and pharyngeal sensory abnormalities in stroke patients with dysphagia. Ann Otol Rhinol Laryngol 1996;105(2):92–7.

23. Donovan NJ, Daniels SK, Edmiaston J, et al. Dysphagia screening: state of the art. Stroke 2013;44(4):e24–31.

24. Walker HK. Cranial nerve XI: the spinal accessory nerve. In: Walker HK, Hall WD, Hurst JW, editors. Clinical methods: the history, physical, and laboratory examinations. 3rd edition. Boston: Butterworths; 1990. Available at: http://www.ncbi.nlm.nih.gov/books/NBK387/. Accessed July 30, 2019.

25. Bamiou DE. Hearing disorders in stroke. Handb Clin Neurol 2015;129:633–47.

26. Leigh RJ, Zee DS. The neurology of eye movements. Oxford: Oxford University Press; 2006.

27. Strupp M, Kremmyda O, Adamczyk C, et al. Central ocular motor disorders, including gaze palsy and nystagmus. J Neurol 2014;261(Suppl 2):542–58.
28. Trobe JD. The neurology of vision. Oxford: Oxford University Press; 2001.
29. Pula JH, Yuen CA. Eyes and stroke: the visual aspects of cerebrovascular disease. Stroke Vasc Neurol 2017;2(4):210–20.
30. Kedar S, Ghate D, Corbett JJ. Visual fields in neuro-ophthalmology. Indian J Ophthalmol 2011;59(2):103–9.
31. Rowe FJ, Wright D, Brand D, et al. A prospective profile of visual field loss following stroke: prevalence, type, rehabilitation, and outcome. Biomed Res Int 2013;2013:719096.
32. Cereda C, Carrera E. Posterior cerebral artery territory infarctions. Front Neurol Neurosci 2012;30:128–31.
33. Terao S, Takatsu S, Izumi M, et al. Central facial weakness due to medial medullary infarction: the course of facial corticobulbar fibres. J Neurol Neurosurg Psychiatry 1997;63(3):391–3.
34. Kumral E, Afsar N, Kirbas D, et al. Spectrum of medial medullary infarction: clinical and magnetic resonance imaging findings. J Neurol 2002;249(1):85–93.
35. Montaner J, Alvarez-Sabín J. Opalski's syndrome. J Neurol Neurosurg Psychiatry 1999;67(5):688–9.
36. Kim BJ, Kang HG, Kim H-J, et al. Magnetic resonance imaging in acute ischemic stroke treatment. J Stroke 2014;16(3):131–45.
37. Williams M. Manual muscle testing, development and current use. Phys Ther Rev 1956;36(12):797–805.
38. Ashizawa T, Xia G. Ataxia. Continuum (MInneap Minn) Lifelong Learn Neurol 2016;22(Movement Disorders):1208–26.
39. Wright J, Huang C, Strbian D, et al. Diagnosis and management of acute cerebellar infarction. Stroke 2014;45(4):e56–8.
40. Gilman S. Joint position sense and vibration sense: anatomical organisation and assessment. J Neurol Neurosurg Psychiatry 2002;73(5):473–7.
41. Becker E, Karnath H-O. Incidence of visual extinction after left versus right hemisphere stroke. Stroke 2007;38(12):3172–4.
42. Bowen A, McKenna K, Tallis RC. Reasons for variability in the reported rate of occurrence of unilateral spatial neglect after stroke. Stroke 1999;30(6):1196–202.
43. Heilman KM, Valenstein E, Watson RT. Neglect and related disorders. Semin Neurol 2000;20(4):463–70.
44. Weintraub S, Mesulam MM. Right cerebral dominance in spatial attention. Further evidence based on ipsilateral neglect. Arch Neurol 1987;44(6):621–5.
45. Ellis SJ, Small M. Denial of illness in stroke. Stroke 1993;24(5):757–9.
46. Damasio AR. Aphasia. N Engl J Med 1992;326(8):531–9.
47. Broca P. Sur le siège de la faculté du langage articulé. Bull Mém Société Anthropol Paris 1865;6(1):377–93.
48. Mohr JP, Pessin MS, Finkelstein S, et al. Broca aphasia: pathologic and clinical. Neurology 1978;28(4):311–24.
49. Wernicke C. Der Aphasische Symptomenkomplex. In: Wernicke C, editor. Der aphasische Symptomencomplex: Eine psychologische Studie auf anatomischer Basis. Berlin: Springer Berlin Heidelberg; 1974. p. 1–70.
50. Wilkins RH, Brody IA. Wernicke's sensory aphasia. Arch Neurol 1970;22(3):279–80.
51. Turkstra L. Fluent aphasia. In: Kreutzer JS, DeLuca J, Caplan B, editors. Encyclopedia of clinical neuropsychology. New York: Springer New York; 2011. p. 1057–9.

# Large Vessel Occlusion in the Acute Stroke Patient

## Identification, Treatment, and Management

Kiffon M. Keigher, MSN, ACNP-BC, RN[a,b,]*

### KEYWORDS

- Acute stroke • Ischemic stroke • Large vessel occlusion
- Mechanical thrombectomy • Intra-arterial thrombolysis • Stent-retriever
- Stroke syndromes • Angiogram

### KEY POINTS

- Stroke is the number 1 disabling disease in the United States and the fifth leading cause of death.
- Early identification of stroke symptoms provides the best opportunity to treat in the early window and minimize disability.
- Large vessel occlusions (LVOs) are often not responsive to IV thrombolysis alone.
- Mechanical thrombectomy procedures should be considered and offered, as indicated, to patients with LVOs up to 24 hours of last known well (LKW).
- Acute stroke care of patients with LVO requires the intensive care nurse to be educated on stroke risk factors, treatment criteria, and postoperative care considerations.

## INTRODUCTION

Acute stroke is a life-threatening disease that remains the major cause of serious disability in the United States.[1] Thus, identification of stroke symptoms as early as possible is critical to patient outcomes. The American Heart Association/American Stroke Association (AHA/ASA) has focused on the FAST acronym for community education on stroke symptom recognition. This acronym stands for the following: F-Face, A-Arm, S-Speech, and T-Time to call 911. The FAST mnemonic is widely accepted as a validated tool. Over the last 6 to 10 years, there has been an explosion of research focused on patients who have an acute occlusion of the large vessels of the brain.

The mainstay of treatment of acute ischemic stroke has been the administration of intravenous (IV) thrombolysis. New trials over the last decade have shown positive

[a] Neurosurgery & Neuroendovascular, Advocate Lutheran General Hospital, Chicago, IL, USA;
[b] Advocate Aurora Health, Chicago, IL, USA
* Advocate Lutheran General Hospital, Center for Advanced Care, 1700 Luther Lane, Park Ridge, IL 60068.
*E-mail address:* kiffon.keigher@advocatehealth.com

Crit Care Nurs Clin N Am 32 (2020) 21–36
https://doi.org/10.1016/j.cnc.2019.11.007
0899-5885/20/© 2019 Elsevier Inc. All rights reserved.

results with treatment of an acute large vessel occlusion (LVO) via a procedure called mechanical thrombectomy. These trials have profoundly changed the management of patients with acute stroke and have had great impact on recovery and outcome.

## EVOLUTION OF STROKE CARE

The spotlight on acute stroke treatment in the last 5 years has expanded, because significant endovascular trials have emphasized the critical nature of the time-dependent intervention of mechanical thrombectomy. The National Institute of Neurologic Disorders and Stroke led the way in pivotal trials that helped prove the safety and efficacy of IV thrombolysis for the treatment of acute stroke. The Food and Drug Administration (FDA) approved the use of Alteplase for acute ischemic strokes in 1996. Initially, thrombolytic therapy was offered to eligible patients up to 4.5 hours from symptom onset.[1] Although IV Alteplase proved to be an effective treatment, it was determined not to be as effective a therapy for patients with LVOs. In 2015, endovascular thrombectomy became the standard of care as a result of 5 randomized control trials (RCTs). These 5 trials, MR CLEAN, ESCAPE, SWIFT PRIME, EXTEND-IA, and REVASCAT, changed the field of neurointervention. These RCTs proved that patients who had thrombectomy with successful recanalization had improved functional outcome scores at 90 days.[2] This was compared with patients who were unable to receive IV thrombolytic therapy, or received IV thrombolytic therapy alone.[2] Two additional landmark trials, DAWN and DEFUSE 3, also demonstrated improved functional outcomes.

Patients meeting eligibility criteria for mechanical thrombectomy had no additional safety risks in the extended window of 16 to 24 hours of last known well (LKW). The ability to offer intervention for LVO beyond the window of 3 to 4.5 hours has provided new treatment options and supportive data demonstrating improved functional outcome scores. Before determining patient eligibility for mechanical thrombectomy, the critical care nurse must first understand the pathology of a large vessel stroke.

## INTRACRANIAL VASCULATURE AND PATHOLOGY OF LARGE VESSEL OCCLUSION

There are 4 major vessels that supply blood flow to the brain: the carotid arteries (right and left) and the vertebral arteries (right and left). The carotid arteries supply most blood flow to the anterior portion of the brain, and the vertebral arteries provide most of the blood flow to the posterior portion of the brain, including the cerebellum.[3] These large vessels branch into smaller intracranial blood vessels forming the Circle of Willis (COW) (**Fig. 1**).

Additional arterial blood supply that contributes to the COW includes the anterior cerebral arteries, the anterior communicating artery, the posterior cerebral arteries, and the posterior communicating arteries. Not all individuals have a complete COW. This is important to understand when we discuss collateral circulation.

An understanding of the cerebrovascular territories assists the bedside nurse to localize the lesion and associated symptoms to the effected vascular area. Localization of the lesion is achieved through highly skilled bedside nursing assessment. This is discussed in depth below.

At stroke onset, LVOs are typically caused by a thrombus (clot) or embolus (moving clot) that becomes lodged into one of the large vessels of the intracranial circulation.[4] When an artery is occluded, that area of the brain becomes hypoperfused, causing diminishing blood flow to meet metabolic demands. The brain has a limited amount of time before cell death occurs and brain tissue becomes ischemic.[4]

It is important to consider the different causes of an LVO and identify a patient's risk factors. Potential causes of stroke, other than thrombus or embolus, include injury to

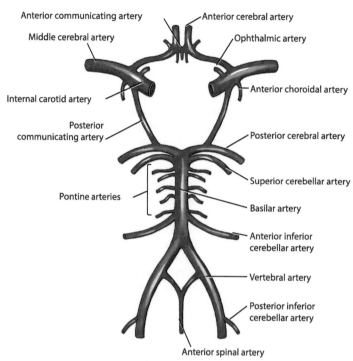

**Fig. 1.** Circle of Willis (COW). (*From* Layne LJ, Petrie L. Vascular, cardiac, and interventional radiography. In: Long BW, Rollins JH, Smith BJ, editors. Merrill's atlas of radiographic positioning and procedures: volume 3, 14th ed. St. Louis: Elsevier; 2019. p. 306; with permission.)

the artery, such as a dissection, which can cause hemodynamic narrowing of the artery.[5] Dissection is a tear of the intima (inner lining) of the artery, causing blood to leak into the media (middle layer) that can cause flow-limiting stenosis (abnormal narrowing) via a true and false lumen of the artery. Blood attempts to fill into the false lumen causing diminished flow in the true lumen needed to perfuse the brain. This high-grade stenosis, or occlusion, can lead to ischemia and stroke. Vasculitis syndromes cause narrowing of the vessels through the release of inflammatory markers that promote vasoconstriction of the arterial wall.[4] These pathological conditions are important to recognize because they often can lead to occlusive disease of the artery putting the patient at increased stroke risk.

Despite having an LVO, some individuals are able to sustain blood flow to the affected area with collateral circulation. Collateral circulation is composed of arterial connections that help to prevent ischemia and infarct. These alternate pathways, or collateral vessels, provide sustained blood flow. Arterial insufficiencies, such as LVO will recruit blood flow from nearby arteries. They work together to preserve brain tissue, and ultimately influence the outcome for the patient. Not all individuals have good collateral circulation, and this is the primary reason behind the variability in stroke outcomes. Individuals with a robust collateral circulation are able to supply needed blood flow for longer periods, whereas others cannot sustain collateral flow for long.[6–8]

Salvageable tissue, known as the penumbra, is brain tissue at risk of evolving to infarct and cell death. Restoration of blood flow via mechanical thrombectomy before the collapse of collateral circulation will be an important determinant of outcome.

## IDENTIFICATION OF LARGE VESSEL OCCLUSION

The influence and role of the first responder to patients with acute stroke cannot be underestimated. This includes physicians, nurses, emergency medical services (EMS), and the community at large. It is essential for health care professionals in the field to recognize that prehospital neuro-assessment, triage, and early transport to an appropriate hospital are key factors in patient outcome. Hospital emergency departments (EDs), in collaboration with stroke and critical care teams, must coordinate efficient workflows to quickly diagnose large vessel strokes and facilitate early intervention in the acute phase. Optimizing workflow to establish earlier recanalization times for a patient from time of symptom onset to time of reperfusion is associated with improved functional patient outcomes.[9,10]

AHA/ASA acute stroke guidelines provide recommendations for prehospital screening. Utilizing an LVO scale provides EMS guidance for triage and transport to the closest stroke center capable of providing the appropriate level of care.[11,12] Although no single LVO tool is yet validated as best practice, a few LVO tools are considered to have good sensitivity and specificity in identification of LVO in the field.

Two of the most common field assessment tools include the Cincinnati Prehospital Stroke Scale (**Fig. 2**) and the Los Angeles Prehospital Stroke Scale (**Fig. 3**). Two of the most commonly used scales in the hospital setting are the Glasgow Coma Scale (GCS) and the National Institutes of Health Stroke Scale (NIHSS). The GCS evaluates eyes, speech, and motor function. The NIHSS is an important tool for critical care clinicians to use and put into practice. This score determines a patient's severity of symptoms and guides eligibility for mechanical thrombectomy procedures. The NIHSS is a scale of 0 to 42 with a higher score indicating a worse clinical examination.

Tools that help in early LVO identification, support rapid triage, and transport to a comprehensive stroke center or thrombectomy-capable hospital that can provide the most appropriate level of care. The importance of early identification is shown to reduce the time of stroke symptom onset to mechanical thrombectomy and subsequent recanalization. In some studies, this has shown to correlate with improved clinical outcomes at 90 days.[13] The meta-analysis of 5 RCTs by Goyal and colleagues,[2] compared functional outcome scores using the modified Rankin Scale (mRS) at

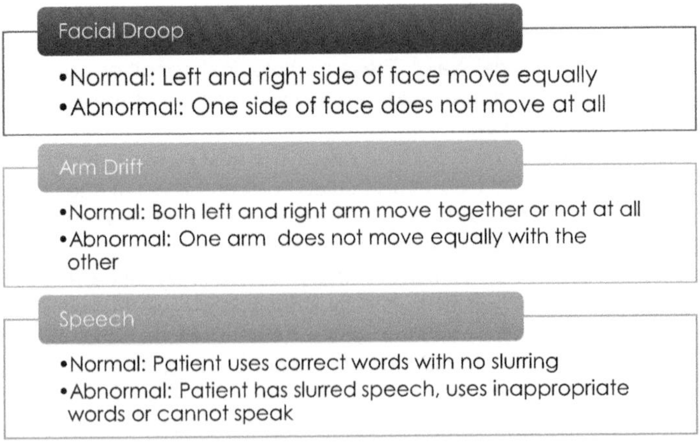

**Facial Droop**
- Normal: Left and right side of face move equally
- Abnormal: One side of face does not move at all

**Arm Drift**
- Normal: Both left and right arm move together or not at all
- Abnormal: One arm does not move equally with the other

**Speech**
- Normal: Patient uses correct words with no slurring
- Abnormal: Patient has slurred speech, uses inappropriate words or cannot speak

**Fig. 2.** Cincinnati prehospital stroke scale. (*Adapted from* Kothari RU, Pancioli A, Liu T, et al. Cincinnati Prehospital Stroke Scale: reproducibility and validity. Ann Emerg Med. 1999;33(4):374; with permission.)

## Los Angeles Prehospital Stroke Screen (LAPSS)

1. Patient Name: _____    _____
   _Last_    _First_

2. Information/History from:
   [ ] Patient
   [ ] Family Member] _____    Phone: _____
   [ ] Other    ⌠ _Name_

3. Last known time patient was at baseline or deficit free and awake:    _Military Time:_ _____
   _Date:_ _____

**SCREENING CRITERIA:**                                          Yes    Unknown    No
4. Age >45                                                        [ ]      [ ]      [ ]
5. History of seizures or epilepsy **absent**                     [ ]      [ ]      [ ]
6. Symptom duration **less than** 24 h                            [ ]      [ ]      [ ]
7. At baseline, patient is **not** wheelchair bound or bedridden  [ ]      [ ]      [ ]

                                                                 Yes              No
8. Blood glucose between 60 and 400:                              [ ]              [ ]

9. Exam: **LOOK FOR OBVIOUS ASYMMETRY**
                          Normal    **Right**          **Left**
   Facial Smile/Grimace:    ☐      ☐ Droop           ☐ Droop

   Grip:                    ☐      ☐ Weak Grip       ☐ Weak Grip
                                   ☐ No Grip         ☐ No Grip

   Arm Strength:            ☐      ☐ Drifts Down     ☐ Drifts Down
                                   ☐ Falls Rapidly   ☐ Falls Rapidly

                                                                 Yes              No
Based on exam, patient has **only unilateral** (and not bilateral) weakness: [ ]   [ ]

10. _**Items 4,5,6,7,8,9 all YES's (or unknown) → LAPSS screening**_    Yes    No
    _**criteria met:**_                                                 [ ]    [ ]

11. If LAPSS criteria for stroke met, call receiving hospital with a "code stroke", if not then return to the appropriate treatment protocol. (Note: the patient may still be experiencing a stroke even if LAPSS criteria are not met.)

**Fig. 3.** Los Angeles prehospital stroke screen. (_From_ Kidwell CS, Starkman S, Eckstein M, et al. Identifying stroke in the field. Prospective validation of the Los Angeles Prehospital Stroke Screen. Stroke 2000;31(1):72; with permission.)

90 days. This analysis compared patients with acute stroke who received mechanical thrombectomy (with or without IV Alteplase) with patients who received IV Alteplase alone, or were ineligible for IV thrombolytic without thrombectomy. Review of the Hermes meta-analysis (**Fig. 4**) showed significant functional improvement at 90 days in the neurointerventional (NIR) treatment arm (with or without IV Alteplase) compared with IV Alteplase, or standard medical arm only. They found that 45% of the interventional treatment arm had good functional status of mRS of 0 to 2 at 90 days compared with only 26% of the IV Alteplase, or standard medical intervention only management group.[2]

Algorithms for field triage, such as the AHA/ASA's Mission: Lifeline Stroke, guide EMS with recommendations for transport to the nearest and most appropriate hospital

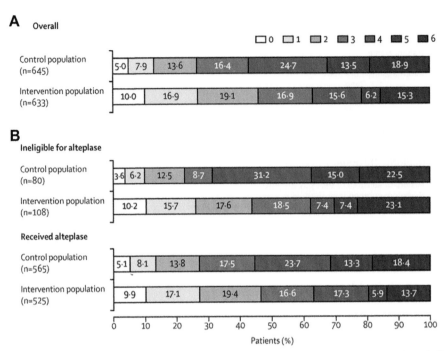

**Fig. 4.** Hermes meta-analysis of 5 randomized control trials (*A*) shows overall results of all patients. (*B*) categorizes the treatment arm of each patient. (*Reprinted with* permission from Elsevier (Goyal M, Menon BK, van Zwam WH, et al. Endovascular thrombectomy after large vessel ischaemic stroke: a meta-analysis of individual patient data from five randomised trials. Lancet 2018;387(10029):1726).

capable of performing mechanical thrombectomy. There are many large vessel screening tools to help identify a patient with LVO in the field. These include Rapid Arterial oCclusion Evaluation, Field Assessment Stroke Triage for Emergency Destination, VAN (Stroke Vision, Aphasia, Neglect Assessment), 3-Item Stroke Scale (3I-SS: 1, level of consciousness; 2, gaze; 3, motor function), and Los Angeles Motor Scale (LAMS) to name a few. LVO scales have variability in elements tested, but focus on positive cortical symptoms in some form, including; weakness, aphasia, neglect, gaze preference, or visual symptoms. Most of these scales demonstrate overall good specificity and sensitivity but no single tool has been validated at this point as the best screening tool to accurately identify LVO (**Table 1**).[10]

## DIAGNOSTIC TESTING FOR DETERMINING THROMBECTOMY ELIGIBILITY

Cerebral vascular imaging is required to diagnose an LVO. The most appropriate imaging to identify an LVO is computed tomography angiography (CTA [vessels]) or magnetic resonance angiography (MRA [vessels]). CTA can be completed with a noncontrast head CT (brain) to rule out hemorrhagic stroke. If CTA or MRA demonstrate evidence of an LVO, the stroke team needs to consider if the patient is eligible for mechanical thrombectomy. The NIR team should already be alerted about the possibility of an acute stroke and possible thrombectomy. The stroke team will begin to prepare the patient either to proceed directly to the angiography lab, or prepare to transfer the patient to a hospital capable of performing mechanical thrombectomy.

**Table 1**
**Large vessel screening tools**

| Scale Name | Examination Components | Score | Sensitivity, % | Specificity, % |
|---|---|---|---|---|
| FAST-ED | • Face weakness<br>• Arm weakness<br>• Speech changes<br>• Gaze<br>• Neglect | ≥4 | 61 | 89 |
| RACE | • Face weakness<br>• Arm weakness<br>• Leg weakness<br>• Gaze<br>• Neglect or aphasia | ≥5 | 85 | 67 |
| 3I-SS | • Level of consciousness<br>• Gaze<br>• Motor weakness | ≥4 | 67 | 92 |
| VAN | • Arm weakness must be present PLUS:<br>• visual disturbance, aphasia, or gaze/neglect | Arm weakness + 1 other positive element | 100 | 90 |
| LAMS | • Face weakness<br>• Arm weakness<br>• Grip | >4 | 81 | 89 |

*Abbreviations:* 3I-SS, 3-item stroke scale; FAST-ED, field assessment stroke triage for emergency destination; LAMS, Los Angeles motor scale; RACE, rapid arterial occlusion evaluation; VAN, stroke vision, aphasia, neglect assessment.
*Data from* Refs.[14–20]

### Eligibility Criteria

The strength of evidence from RCTs has provided a framework of eligibility criteria for mechanical thrombectomy. It should be noted that these trials provide recommendations, although clinical judgment remains a key component in determining if a patient should be offered mechanical thrombectomy. Criteria include, but are not limited to:[6,7,11]

- Confirmed LVO on vascular imaging (ICA, M1, basilar artery)
- Baseline mRS of 0 to 2
- NIHSS ≥6, or disabling deficit, such as aphasia
- LKW less than 24 hours
- Evidence of salvageable brain tissue on CT or MR perfusion imaging (ie, good mismatch)
- Small core infarct (per DAWN/DEFUSE3 criteria) on CT or MR perfusion imaging
- Suspicion for posterior circulation stroke (ie, basilar artery occlusion)

Patients presenting with stroke symptoms, without evidence of an LVO on vascular imaging would not qualify for thrombectomy given no evidence of a clot to treat. Patients who have multiple comorbid conditions and poor functional ability at baseline or those with a life-threatening disease with limited life expectancy are unlikely to benefit. Patients who arrive 24 hours after LKW with an anterior circulation LVO do not meet thrombectomy criteria due to the increased risk of potential bleeding and lack of benefit. Finally, patients with a large territory infarct, and small mismatch, will not be eligible for acute therapy. Identifying patients who have contraindications for thrombectomy is important in the prevention of potential reperfusion hemorrhage, and the risk of a procedure that may provide no benefit.

Current trials are continuing to re-evaluate eligibility criteria. Examples include studies looking at outcomes of patients with LVO undergoing thrombectomy with low NIHSS score or with large core infarcts. Results of these new trials would potentially provide evidence to further expand acute interventions to a larger population of stroke patients.

## ANGIOGRAM AND MECHANICAL THROMBECTOMY

A cerebral angiogram provides images of blood vessels in and around the brain. The gold standard remains the conventional digital subtraction angiography. Conventional angiography is the only method by which a trained neurointerventionalist can perform a thrombectomy procedure. Mechanical thrombectomy is an intervention where a catheter is introduced into the artery, most common the femoral artery, and navigated to the artery of occlusion. From here, the interventionalist will choose from a few devices to mechanically "snare or grab" the clot and retrieve the clot from the artery. Some commonly used devices in this procedure include aspiration catheters and stent-retrievers. The number of attempts needed to snare a clot varies by provider. Ideally, the clot is retrieved on a first pass with minimal disruption to the endothelial wall of the artery and early recanalization of the vessel is achieved, restoring blood flow.

The goals of achieving recanalization are varied but the AHA/ASA has set primary goals in Target: Stroke Phase III.[21] These guidelines recommend from door to first pass (of thrombectomy device) within 90 minutes for direct arriving patients, and within 60 minutes for transfers. The aim is to achieve this goal in greater than 50% of acute stroke patients with LVO treated with mechanical endovascular therapy.[21]

The scale used to evaluate reperfusion efficacy is the Thrombolysis in Cerebral Infarction (TICI) scale. This measures the extent of perfusion using a grading scale of TICI 0 to 3 (**Table 2**). All endovascular trials since 2015 have identified good functional outcomes as mRS of 0 to 2, with quality reperfusion of at least TICI 2b or 3. Reperfusion quality less than TICI 2b is a predictor of poor functional outcome for patients at 90 days.[22] It is important for clinicians caring for stroke patients to understand the meaning of this scale. It identifies the quality of reperfusion of the brain

| Table 2 | |
|---------|---|
| **Modified thrombolysis in cerebral infarction scale** | |
| **TICI Grade** | **TICI Defined** |
| 0 | No perfusion to the identified territory |
| 1 | Minimal perfusion |
| 2a | Partial perfusion that is filling <50% of the of the occluded arteries identified territory |
| 2b | Partial perfusion that is filling >50% of the of the occluded arteries identified territory |
| 3 | Complete reperfusion of identified territory |

[a]Based on angiographic appearance of the occluded blood vessel.

*Data from* Fugate JE, Klunder AM, Kallmes DF. What is meant by "TICI"? ANJR Am J Neuroradiol. 2013;34(9):1792–7.

after thrombectomy. For those patients after thrombectomy with a TICI of 0, 1, or 2a we can expect disability that is more serious and a poor outcome.[23] This may help guide family discussions and further medical decision-making options for the patient.

## STROKE WORKFLOWS

Early notification of the interventional neuroradiology team is crucial to timely reperfusion. As discussed, time goals from door to puncture, first pass of device, and recanalization times are established goals for the team to achieve. Creation of stroke workflows for thrombectomy-eligible patients is important to achieve set goals. Hospitals providing mechanical thrombectomy will have varied algorithms for team members (**Fig. 5**), but all provide a framework for role delineation and a stepwise process by which patient eligibility and flow from the ED to the angiography lab is determined.

## NEUROLOGIC EXAMINATION AND ASSESSMENT

The ability to identify an LVO requires an understanding of the basic functions of brain anatomy and vascular territories. As previously noted, stroke symptoms provide specific clues to the affected vascular territory. Symptoms of LVO of the anterior circulation, including carotids and/or middle cerebral arteries, will often be quite different from those of an occluded artery of the posterior circulation, such as the basilar artery. Although we cannot review all stroke syndromes here, **Table 3** helps identify common symptoms associated with LVO.[24]

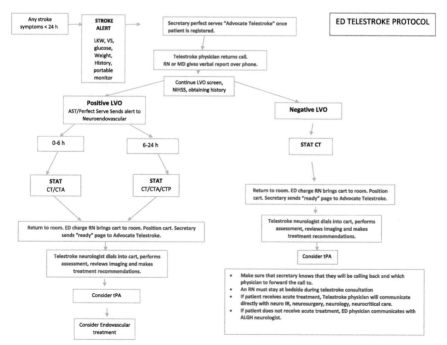

**Fig. 5.** Comprehensive stroke center stroke alert workflow from Advocate Lutheran General Hospital.

**Table 3**
**Large vessel occlusion and associated symptoms and syndromes**

| Occluded Vessel | Anterior Circulation | | Other Considerations |
|---|---|---|---|
| | **Dominant** | **Nondominant** | |
| Internal carotid artery | • Aphasia<br>• Contralateral homonymous hemianopsia<br>• Contralateral motor and sensory loss of face, arm, and leg | • Neglect<br>• Contralateral homonymous hemianopsia<br>• Contralateral motor and sensory loss of face, arm, and leg | • *Horner's syndrome* can be seen with carotid dissection—ptosis (droopiness of eyelid), miosis (pupillary constriction) and anhidrosis (decreased sweating)<br>• *Amaurosis fugax*—transient monocular blindness often described as a "shade" pulled down over the eye"<br>• *Central retinal artery occlusion (CRAO)*—sudden loss of vision in 1 eye, painless |
| Middle cerebral artery | • Aphasia<br>• Contralateral hemiparesis (arm more than leg)<br>• Contralateral sensory loss<br>• Eye (gaze) deviation toward the affected side<br>• Homonymous hemianopia | • Neglect<br>• Contralateral hemiparesis (arm more than leg)<br>• Contralateral sensory loss<br>• Eye (gaze) deviation toward the affected side | • Hemiparesis in this territory most often affects the arm more than the leg<br>• Neglect syndromes can include: anosognosia |

| Posterior Circulation | Symptoms | Identified Syndromes |
|---|---|---|
| Vertebral artery | • Dizziness<br>• Diplopia<br>• Contralateral hemiparesis<br>• Contralateral hemisensory loss<br>• Ataxic motor<br>• Ataxic gait | • *Lateral medullary syndrome (Wallenberg syndrome* —ipsilateral sensory loss of face, ipsilateral ataxia, contralateral hemisensory loss of pain and temperature, vertigo |
| Basilar artery | • Ataxic hemiparesis<br>• Dysconjugate gaze<br>• Mixed motor examination (bilateral and/or waxing and waning weakness), quadriparesis<br>• Altered mental status and level of consciousness<br>• Cranial nerve deficits<br>• Dysarthria<br>• Coma | • *Locked-in syndrome*—weakness of UE and LE and face, loss of speech or severe dysarthria, lateral gaze weakness<br>• *Ventral pontine syndrome (Millard-Gubler syndrome)*—contralateral weakness of UE/LE, lateral gaze weakness, diplopia, ipsilateral facial weakness |

*Abbreviations:* LE, lower extremity; UE, upper extremity.
[a]Dominant hemisphere (left side); nondominant (right side).
*Data from* Pare JR, Kahn JH. Basic neuroanatomy and stroke syndromes. Emerg Med Clin North Am. 2012;30(3):601–615.

## PREOPERATIVE CARE AND CONSIDERATIONS

In preparation for an angiogram procedure, it is important for the critical care nurse to be thinking about key assessment pieces. **Table 4** identifies key diagnostic and examination considerations for the nurse to complete before the angiogram procedure. Completion of a neurologic assessment, review of diagnostics, and providing education are important elements to complete before bringing the patient to the angiography lab. Informed consent is required for all procedures and surgeries. Although mechanical thrombectomy is the standard of care and should be offered to all eligible patients, providers should follow their hospital protocols and policies for medical necessity documentation with regard to emergent procedures in the absence of decisional capacity or a surrogate family member.

## INTRAPROCEDURAL CONSIDERATIONS

The procedural nurse should consider and anticipate special needs of the stroke patient undergoing mechanical thrombectomy. Common procedural considerations include, monitoring the ABCs (airway, breathing, circulation). Is the patient protecting their airway?

| Table 4 Nursing considerations preparing for mechanical thrombectomy | |
|---|---|
| Diagnostic tests | *Imaging:* CT head and CTA head/neck and CT perfusion (if indicated in window greater than 6 h) *Labwork:* glucose, creatinine, hemoglobin, platelet count, PT/INR and PTT most critical *Pregnancy test:* POC if will not delay procedure |
| Vital signs | Stable? Baseline cardiac rhythm? Atrial fibrillation? Baseline blood pressure? Oxygenating and protecting airway? |
| Allergies | Contrast allergy will require premedication |
| Informed consent | If no family present and patient unable to consent self, medical necessity note for thrombectomy is needed |
| Patient tolerance | Can patient tolerate laying flat and still without sedation? |
| Antiplatelets or anticoagulants | Is patient currently taking anticoagulants or antiplatelets? When was last dose? What is the indication? |
| NPO Status | Identify last meal time if able |
| Assessments | *Physical examination:* include a cardiac and carotid assessment (atrial fibrillation, bruit) and a peripheral vascular assessment before arterial puncture *Neurologic examination:* perform a thorough neurologic examination before procedure *NIHSS:* score before going to thrombectomy |
| Team members | Are all team members present to be able to proceed to angiography lab? |
| Education | Educate patient, if appropriate, and family about the angiogram procedure for thrombectomy |
| Time and goals of reperfusion | Note the time of arrival and last known well and set a clock to meet reperfusion goals |

*Abbreviations:* POC, point of care; PT/INR, prothrombin time/international normalized ratio; PTT, partial thromboplastin time.

Is oxygenation adequate (SpO$_2$ > 94%)?[9] Is hypertension or hypotension an issue? What are the procedure blood pressure (BP) goals? BP goals depend on variables, such as patient baseline BP or if they received IV thrombolysis. After Alteplase administration, BP management is required according to post thrombolytic guidelines (<180/105 mm Hg for the first 24 hours).[9] Hypertension is allowed in the setting of LVO, and without IV thrombolytic administration, until reperfusion is achieved. Identify if there is evidence of an abnormal heart rhythm that may require immediate intervention (atrial fibrillation with rapid ventricular response) The use of general anesthesia versus conscious sedation varies among hospitals and is typically done according to provider preference.

Also important to consider are potential allergies to iodine-based contrast or other procedural medications. IV administration of steroids and antihistamines are indicated for those patients with known or suspected iodine allergy. Close monitoring for anaphylaxis and the need for intubation is a priority.

Tandem occlusions of the cervical internal carotid artery are becoming more common, with increased volume of intervention, and expanded indications for LVO treatment. A tandem occlusion is an occlusion of a carotid artery on the ipsilateral (same) side as the occluded intracranial vessel. Thrombus and occlusion of the carotid artery in these cases are thought to be the culprit for stroke mechanism. For this reason, tandem occlusions are often treated acutely with carotid stenting at the time of mechanical thrombectomy. The placement of a stent in the parent vessel of an artery requires the initiation of an antiplatelet medication to prevent stent thrombosis. For those patients who have received IV thrombolytic therapy, mechanical thrombectomy, and carotid stenting, the risk for hemorrhage increases. Close monitoring is a nursing priority. This situation has become so frequent that the 2019 Guidelines for Acute Ischemic Stroke have made new recommendations on antiplatelets to avoid, and alternative medications to consider in this particular setting.[11] The use of IV antiplatelets[9] followed by oral medications, such as aspirin and/or clopidogrel, are common in this setting.

## POSTOPERATIVE CARE FOR MECHANICAL THROMBECTOMY

The nursing care post thrombectomy focuses primarily on BP goals, neurologic assessment, assessment of the arterial puncture site, monitoring for malignant cerebral edema, and general critical care issues and concerns in the critically ill patient.

### Blood Pressure

It is important to confirm, with the NIR team, successful recanalization of TICI 2b or 3. This will help to make decisions for appropriate BP goals. Establishing defined BP parameters for the stroke patient after LVO reperfusion is imperative. It is clear that the patient with a recent stroke needs to have adequate blood perfusion to the brain. It is also understood that if thrombectomy was successful in achieving TICI 2b or 3 then the patient now has complete, or almost complete, filling of that vascular territory. Because the blood-brain barrier may be impaired from the pathophysiologic state of the ischemic penumbra, it is important to prevent reperfusion hemorrhage. This is a balance that must be considered when establishing BP parameters for the post thrombectomy patient. This practice varies widely among interventionalists. Recent guidelines recommend maintaining BP between 120 and 160 mm Hg as a reasonable target for those patients with TICI 2b or 3 recanalization.[25,26] For patients who do not achieve TICI 2b or 3 recanalization, a higher BP is indicated. Literature supports allowing systolic BP up to 220 without IV thrombolytics or less than 180 after thrombolytics.[25]

*Arterial Puncture Site*
___

It is important to perform a preoperative assessment of the puncture site and baseline peripheral vascular assessments. Baseline assessments help to easily identify new findings or potential complications post procedure. It is common for the neurointerventionalist to use the femoral artery for access, but may also use radial artery access or another approach. Skin color and temperature, capillary refill, and pulse checks are critical for the patient who has had an arterial sheath placed. In addition, monitoring for swelling at the site, drainage from the site, or any pain, numbness, or tingling in the extremity is important to identify early complications.

Complications to consider specific to arterial access site:

- Hematoma of the arterial access puncture site: monitor for swelling and/or bleeding at the site; application of manual pressure for at least 30 minutes is indicated
- Retroperitoneal hematoma: most often associated with hypotension, low back pain, and difficulties voiding; will also see a drop in hemoglobin; prepare for volume resuscitation and/or blood transfusion
- Occlusion of the artery: occlusion of the punctured artery may be a vascular emergency, particularly if it is the femoral artery; thorough peripheral vascular assessments are critical, emergent vascular consult indicated if loss of pulse and cold extremity
- Arterial injury of the punctured blood vessel: pseudoaneurysms or fistulas may result if there is an injury to the punctured artery; lower extremity duplex can confirm this finding, thrombin injection is a rarely needed intervention for small pseudoaneurysms

*Neurologic Assessments*
___

It is imperative to provide a thorough neurologic examination. Nursing clinical assessment skills can help identify, in the early stages, potential problems, complications post procedure, or new issues from evolving stroke infarct, or reperfusion hemorrhage. Red flags would include new onset or severe headache, nausea, or any change in neurologic examination. For patients with an LVO and large stroke burden, there should be a low threshold for obtaining a rapid head CT scan for any neurologic examination change, due to the potential for increasing cerebral edema or bleed. Goals of care for the patient are important to establish early with the family if the patient is unable to participate in establishing goals for themselves.

Other complications to consider post procedure:

- Hemorrhagic conversion or other bleeding: sudden onset headaches or altered mental status is warning sign and CT head should be performed immediately; monitoring of other sites for bleeding
- Reocclusion of artery: change or worsening in neurologic examination could indicate vessel reocclusion or a new occlusion of a different artery
- Malignant cerebral edema: most common with middle cerebral artery occlusions; can consider hemicraniectomy; discussion of risk/benefit and anticipated prognosis between family and neurosurgery team

Finally, we need to consider the patient's medical risk factors and controlling acute issues we commonly see in our critically ill population.[3,9] Medical management considerations include:

- Initiation of antiplatelet therapy (ie, aspirin)
- Glucose control

- Cholesterol management and initiation of a high dose statin if not contraindicated
- Targeted temperature management
- Deep venous thrombosis prevention and prophylaxis
- Swallow evaluations and aspiration precautions
- Nutritional status
- Early rehabilitation
- Positioning and mobilization of body and limbs
- Stroke education
- Holistic care and counseling when indicated

## NEW HORIZONS

Neuroendovascular intervention and stroke research is expanding, new devices, artificial intelligence (AI), field triage recommendations, and robotic technology are on the forefront. We are seeing Health Insurance Portability and Accountability Act-compliant mobile apps (Allm, Inc, Japan) assisting in real-time communication and sharing of digital imaging and communications in medicine. These customizable chat groups are favored by acute stroke teams allowing for easier communication between team members in "real" time and collaboration of tasks.[27] Imaging software algorithms, such as RAPID (iSchemaView) provide fast, automated imaging results for early clinical decision-making for stroke care providers.[6] Other cutting-edge technologies being evaluated have the capability of detecting vasospasm with wearable helmets (NeuralAnalytics, Los Angeles). This technology provides early diagnostics without the need for conventional imaging. The US FDA-approved AI applications, such as that provided by Viz.ai, Inc (Tel Aviv), capable of early identification of LVO and virtual reality platforms to aid in rehabilitation. New AI with automated notification systems provide early identification of LVO or hemorrhage on CT and CTA before patients even leave the CT scanners.

Advances in technology and devices are aimed at improving the efficiency and speed of stroke care triage with the promise of early treatment of a patient with an LVO. The full impact of this new technology and supporting research is still to be determined. Initial feedback seems to have positive influence on stroke team workflows and with improved ease of early identification and treatment of patients with LVO.

## SUMMARY

Treatment options for acute stroke remain time dependent. Patients meeting eligibility criteria with an identified LVO should be offered treatment with mechanical thrombectomy up to 24 hours of LKW. This requires early identification by first responders, efficient triage, and transport to an advanced comprehensive stroke center. The critical care, ED, and NIR teams must collaborate for early door to groin puncture times, allowing for early reperfusion of the brain. We now know patients who achieve early recanalization have the best opportunity for meaningful recovery, good functional outcome, and return to a quality life.

## DISCLOSURE

The author has nothing to disclose.

## REFERENCES

1. Benjamin EJ, Virani SS, Callaway CW, et al, on behalf of the American Heart Association Statistics Committee and Stroke Statistics Subcommittee. Heart disease

and stroke statistics—2018 update: a report from the American Heart Association. Circulation 2018;137:e67–492.

2. Goyal M, Menon BK, van Zwam WH, et al. Endovascular thrombectomy after large vessel ischaemic stroke: a meta-analysis of individual patient data from five randomised trials. Lancet 2018;387(10029):1723–31.

3. Haines DE. Anatomical-clinical correlations: cerebral angiogram, MRA, and MRV. In: Neuroanatomy: an atlas of structures, sections and systems. 7th edition. Philadelphia: Lippincott Williams & Wilkins; 2008. p. 265–77.

4. Livesay S. Anatomy and physiology. In: Livesay S, editor. Comprehensive review for stroke nursing. 1st edition. Chicago: American Association of Neuroscience Nurses; 2014. p. 1–18.

5. Boehme AK, Esenwa C, Elkind MS. Stroke risk factors, genetics, and prevention. Circ Res 2017;120:472–95.

6. Albers GW, Marks MP, Kemp S, et al, for the DEFUSE 3 Investigators. Thrombectomy for stroke at 6 to 16 hours with selection by perfusion imaging. N Engl J Med 2018;378:708–18.

7. Nogueira RG, Jadhav AP, Haussen DC, et al, for the DAWN Trial Investigators. Thrombectomy 6 to 24 hours after stroke with a mismatch between deficit and infarct. N Engl J Med 2018;378:11–21.

8. Stroke statistics. Centers for Disease Control and Prevention. Available at: www.cdc.gov/stroke/. Accessed May 17, 2019.

9. Schregel K, Behme D, Tsogkas I, et al. Effects of workflow optimization in endovascularly treated stroke patients-a pre-post effectiveness study. J Vis Exp 2018;(131):e56397.

10. Ver Hage A, Teleb M, Smith E. An emergent large vessel occlusion screening protocol for acute stroke: a quality improvement initiative. J Neurosci Nurs 2018; 50(2):68–73.

11. Powers WJ, Rabinstein AA, Ackerson T, et al, on behalf of the American Heart Association Stroke Council. Guidelines for the early management of patients with acute ischemic stroke: 2019 update to the 2018 Guidelines for the early management of acute ischemic stroke. Stroke 2019. https://doi.org/10.1161/STR. 0000000000000211.

12. Marini C, De Santis F, Sacco S, et al. Contribution of atrial fibrillation to incidence and outcome of ischemic stroke: results from a population based study. Stroke 2005;36:1115–9.

13. Ng YS, Stein J, Ning M, et al. Comparison of clinical characteristics and functional outcomes of ischemic stroke in different vascular territories. Stroke 2007;38: 2309–14.

14. Schieb LJ, Casper ML, George MG. Mapping primary and comprehensive stroke centers by certification organization. Circ Cardiovasc Qual Outcomes 2015;8: S193–4.

15. Fugate JE, Klunder AM, Kallmes DF. What is meant by "TICI". AJNR Am J Neuroradiol 2013;34(9):1792–7.

16. Teleb MS, Ver Hage A, Carter J, et al. Stroke, vision, aphasia, neglect (VAN) assessment - a novel emergent large vessel screening tool: pilot study and comparison with current clinical severity indices. J Neurointerv Surg 2017;9:122–6.

17. Carrera D, Gorchs M, Querol M, et al, on behalf of the Catalan Stroke Code and Reperfusion Consortium (Cat-SCR). Revalidation of the RACE scale after its regional implementation in Catalonia: a triage tool for large vessel occlusion. J Neurointerv Surg 2019;11:751–6.

18. Lima FO, Silva GS, Furie KL, et al. Field assessment stroke triage for emergency destination. Stroke 2016;47:1997–2002.
19. Gupta R, Manuel M, Owada K, et al. Severe hemiparesis as a prehospital tool to triage stroke severity: a pilot study to assess diagnostic accuracy and treatment times. J Neurointerv Surg 2016;8:775–7.
20. Keenan KJ, Kircher C, McMullan JT. Prehospital prediction of large vessel occlusion in suspected stroke patients. Curr Atheroscler Rep 2018;20:34.
21. American Heart Association. Target: stroke phase III. 2018. Available at: www.heart.org/en/professional/quality-improvement/target-stroke/introducing-target-stroke-phase-ii. Accessed May 28, 2019.
22. Kaesmacher J, Dobrocky T, Heldner MR, et al. Systematic review and meta-analysis on outcome differences among patients with TICI2b versus TICI3 reperfusions: success revisited. J Neurol Neurosurg Psychiatry 2018;89:910–7.
23. Rangaraju S, Haussen D, Nogueira R, et al. Comparison of 3-month stroke disability and quality of life across the modified Rankin scale categories. Interv Neurol 2017;6(1–2):36–41.
24. Pare JR, Kahn JH. Basic neuroanatomy and stroke syndromes. Emerg Med Clin North Am 2012;30(3):601–15.
25. Jadhav AP, Molyneaux BJ, Hill MD, et al. Care of the post thrombectomy patient. Stroke 2018;49:2801–7.
26. Mokin M, Ansari SA, McTaggart RA, et al. Indications for thrombectomy in acute ischemic stroke from emergent large vessel occlusion (ELVO): report of the SNIS standards and guidelines committee. J Neurointerv Surg 2019;11:215–20.
27. Munich SA, Tan LA, Nogueira DM, et al. Mobile real-time tracking of acute stroke patients and instant secure inter-team communication—the JOIN app. Neurointervention 2017;12(2):69–76.

# Cryptogenic Stroke
## Anatomy of the Stroke Work-Up

Mary P. Amatangelo, DNP, RN, ACNP-BC, CCRN, CNRN, SCRN, FAHA

## KEYWORDS

- Cryptogenic stroke • Embolic Stroke of Undetermined Etiology (ESUS)
- Ischemic stroke • Diagnostic testing • Cardiac monitoring • Hypercoagulable
- Imaging

## KEY POINTS

- There are a variety of stroke definitions, advancements in diagnostic technologies, differing thoughts on appropriate etiologic investigations, and more than 200 known causes of ischemic stroke (IS) requiring elimination.
- It is important to determine the cause of cryptogenic stroke (CS) to understand the functional prognosis and eliminate the risk of stroke recurrence by providing appropriate secondary stroke prevention.
- In clinical practice, the diagnosis of CS is considered, when the diagnostic assessment is not complete, when a single cause cannot be determined for there are several potential causes, or there is no identifiable cause despite an extensive evaluation.

## INTRODUCTION

The diagnosis of cryptogenic stroke (CS) is made by exclusion. There are a variety of stroke definitions, advancements in diagnostic technologies, along with differing thoughts on appropriate etiologic investigations, and there are more than 200 known causes of ischemic stroke (IS) requiring elimination.[1] Despite an extensive evaluation the cause of CS cannot be determined in 30% to 40% of cases.[2] It is important to determine the cause of CS to understand the functional prognosis and eliminate the risk of stroke recurrence by providing appropriate secondary stroke prevention.

In clinical practice, the diagnosis of CS is considered when the diagnostic assessment is not complete, when a single cause cannot be determined because there are several potential causes, or there is no identifiable cause despite an extensive evaluation.[5]

Understanding stroke subtype is essential for managing acute interventions and secondary prevention. One prominently used classification system, designed for the TRIAL of ORG-10172 for Acute Stroke Treatment (TOAST), defined an undetermined stroke as a "brain infarction that is not attributable to a cardio-embolic source, large

Neurology, Stroke, Neurocritical Care, Brigham and Women's Hospital, 15 Francis Street, BB 335, Boston, MA 02115, USA
E-mail address: MAMATANGELO@BWH.HARVARD.EDU

Crit Care Nurs Clin N Am 32 (2020) 37–50
https://doi.org/10.1016/j.cnc.2019.11.008
0899-5885/20/© 2019 Elsevier Inc. All rights reserved.

ccnursing.theclinics.com

> **Stroke Mechanism**
>
> Thrombotic (20%)[3]
> - Arterial plaque as a result of atherosclerosis
>
> Cardioembolic (20%)
> - Blood clot from faulty heart valve or atrial fibrillation (AF)
> - Results when a clot dislodges and travels to an area of decreased circulation
>
> Lacunar (25%)
> - Small-vessel disease
> - A vessel is coated with a lipid compound, a process known as lipohyalinosis, which causes the lumen to thicken and restricts blood flow
> - Associated with hypertension
>
> Cryptogenic (30%)
> - No cause found for stroke
>
> Other (5%)
> - Coagulopathies
> - Vasculitis
> - Drug abuse
> - Infections[4]

artery atherosclerosis, or small-vessel disease, despite an extensive vascular, cardiac and serologic evaluation."[5] As such, the definition is thought of in negative terms, based on the absence of findings.

> **TOAST classification of acute IS denotes five subtypes[5]:**
>
> - Large-artery atherosclerosis (thrombosis/embolus)[a]
>   - Carotid/vertebral, intracranial/extracranial, aortic arch
>   - Stenosis, dissection, vasculitis
> - Cardioembolism (high risk/medium risk)[a]
>   - AFib, dilated cardiomyopathy, patent foramen ovale (PFO), endocarditis
> - Small-vessel occlusion (lacune)[a]
>   - Hypertension
> - Stroke of other determined etiology[a]
>   - Hypercoagulable states, iatrogenic, carotid/vertebral dissection
> - Stroke of undetermined cause
>   - Two or more causes identified
>   - Negative evaluation
>   - Incomplete evaluation

## EMBOLIC STROKE OF UNDETERMINED SOURCE (ESUS)

Another definition, based on infarct topography,[6] is the inference being that all nonlacunar IS are caused by embolism.[7] In 2014, the clinical construct of embolic stroke of undetermined source (ESUS) was introduced to identify patients with nonlacunar CS in whom embolism was the likely stroke mechanism.[8]

---

[a] Possible or probably depending on results of ancillary studies.

The main rationale for such an approach has been to define this group of patients in a positive manner, to enable a clearer definition for conduct of randomized controlled trials, and by extension, implications for clinical practice. Developing a consensus definition for CS requires agreement on what is considered to be an extensive or adequate evaluation and which findings are considered etiologic (**Box 1**).[9]

---

**Box 1**
**Criteria for diagnosis of Embolic Stroke of Undetermined Source (ESUS)**

1. IS detected by computed tomography or MRI that is not lacunar

2. Absence of extracranial or intracranial atherosclerosis causing greater than 50% luminal stenosis in arteries supplying the area of ischemia

3. No major risk of cardioembolic source of embolism

4. No other specific cause of stroke identified (eg, arteritis, dissection, migraine/vasospasm, and drug abuse)[10]

---

## INDIVIDUAL RISK FACTORS
### Age

A patient's age is indicative to the likelihood of a variety of stroke causes. In young adults 18 to 30 years of age, dissection is the most common, but congenital cardiac disease and thrombophilia are also notable causes. In those 31 to 60 years of age, early onset atherosclerosis and acquired structural cardiac diseases are increasingly common. As the population ages, the likelihood of specific stroke subtypes is also expected to change. In patients older than 60 years of age, occult atrial fibrillatin (AFib) becomes more frequent.[11] AFib is the most common source of cardiogenic embolism, and increases from 1.5% in 50 to 59 year olds to 23.5% in those aged 80 to 89 years.[12] Understanding the changing patterns of stroke subtypes is important for anticipating the appropriate allocation of preventive and treatment resources and their cost implications for the health care system.[13]

### Medical History

The evaluation of a patient with IS should include a careful history regarding symptom onset, progression, associated symptoms, and medical history. A history of neck injury and headache at the time of onset can suggest dissection as a cause, and associated palpitations or chest pain might suggest a cardioembolic source.[14] Patients should be screened for modifiable risk factors: hypertension, diabetes (by serum glucose or hemoglobin $A_{1C}$), hyperlipidemia (by serum lipids), heart disease (ASCVD calculator), obesity (body mass index [BMI]), smoking (PPD x years), and excessive alcohol use (drinks per day per week).[15]

### Comorbidities and In-hospital Stays

In-hospital strokes are considered a complication of an illness that resulted during a hospitalization, or an iatrogenic consequence related to the withdrawal of a protective therapy (anticoagulation), or of therapeutic interventions during hospitalization. Common mechanisms may be related to a direct complication of vessel manipulation (catheterization), brain ischemia from systemic hypoperfusion (an occluded or suboc-clusive vessel, hypotension), or a thromboembolic event (deep vein thrombosis [DVT], cancer, stroke), or caused by stasis (bedrest) along with events induced by comorbid illness or surgery.[16] Underlying risks may be increased by withdrawal of antithrombotic or anticoagulant therapy because of bleeding, inability to take oral medications, or invasive procedures. Hospitalized patients may experience any combination of these factors, which may help to explain the increase in risk for stroke in patients hospitalized compared with those in the community.[17]

## Baseline Stroke Work-Up

Stroke patients admitted to the intensive care unit (ICU) typically have an initial work-up completed in the emergency department (ED), or at an outside hospital (OSH) prior to transfer. Hence, stroke patients arriving to the ICU often present with a presumed initial stroke diagnosis.

Patients transferred for ICU care from an OSH should arrive with documentation of the initial evaluation, including presenting symptoms, laboratory results, and care provided, along with imaging done prior to transfer (imaging on disk should accompany transferred patients) to avoid repetition of studies. If a patient received intravenous (IV) alteplase prior to arrival, drug bolus and infusion dosage, along with time initiated, should be clearly documented. Approximately 15% to 20% of patients with IS will require care in an ICU.[18]

There is no agreement about the baseline clinical investigation of CS, but recent studies note the investigation should include obtaining a brain computed tomography (CT) or magnetic resonance imaging (MRI) of the brain, 12-lead EKG, cardiac monitoring for 24 hours (Holter), transthoracic echocardiogram (TTE), screening for a prothrombotic (hypercoagulable) state in patients younger than 55 years, CT angiography (CTA) or MRI angiography (MRA) or cervical and intracranial digital angiography, and ultrasonography (US) Doppler of cervical and vertebral arteries.[19,20]

## Neuroimaging

The initial evaluation of patients with suspected stroke includes a head CT without contrast. Head CT is widely available, rapidly obtained, and less expensive than other imaging modalities, such as brain (MRI), although not as sensitive detecting small infarcts that may be important to characterize stroke mechanism. Although CT and MRI have the same sensitivity in excluding hemorrhage, brain MRI is superior to CT in detecting acute infarction.[20–22]

The topographic characteristics of stroke (infarct location and volume) are determined by brain MRI, including diffusion sequences (DWI and ADC), which are more sensitive to small lesions (lesions in the cerebellum and brainstem). These topographic features provide important etiologic information, such as infarcts in multiple brain territories suggest emboli from a proximal aortocardiac source; infarcts of different ages in a single territory suggest emboli of arterial origin; infarcts along the borders between brain artery territories suggest systemic hypotension or multiple emboli; and a small, deep infarct along with white-matter hyperintensities suggests intrinsic small-vessel disease.[11]

Intracranial (brain) and cervical (neck) vasculature (vessels) are investigated by MRA (vessels), CTA (vessels), or digital subtraction angiography (fluoroscopy). Time of flight (TOF) MRA (uses a measure of blood flow as opposed to contrast) and may exaggerate the degree of stenosis in comparison with CTA or carotid ultrasound (US) (decreased flow may give the impression of a decreased lumen caliber). If MRA and CTA are not available (or contraindicated), the carotid arteries are assessed with Doppler Ultrasound (US) to look for stenosis or dissection.[15]

## Cardiac Monitoring

A single electrocardiogram (EKG) is not likely to detect AFib or flutter in 24 hours of cardiac telemetry.[23] Outpatient cardiac monitoring for occult AFib is now the standard of care after CS, for the detection of AFib leads to initiating anticoagulation therapy that is superior to antiplatelet therapy.[24] Studies have shown that the longer patients are monitored, the more likely AFib will be detected.[25] There is a chance, however, that some of the AFib detected may not be causative of the stroke event.

The most cost-effective approach to cardiac monitoring has yet to be determined. It may be prudent to begin with noninvasive 30-day cardiac monitoring initially, especially in patients with a high index of suspicion for AFib, and a high likelihood of compliance with 30-day monitoring. An unrevealing 30-day monitor does not exclude the presence of AFib, and these patients should be considered to undergo an implantable cardiac monitor for longer monitoring.[26]

The heart should be assessed by TTE to evaluate for thrombus, left atrial dilatation (which may be associated with AFib), and valvular vegetation (although transesophageal echocardiogram [TEE] is more sensitive to assess for vegetation).[15] Several studies have shown TTE and perhaps TEE are useful in identifying a potential cardiac source in patients with CS.[14]

An agitated saline (bubble) study is done during the TTE to look for patent foramen ovale (PFO), typically in those aged less than 65. If a PFO is found, a search for deep vein thrombosis (DVT) is undertaken with Doppler US of the lower extremities, and pelvic MR venography to evaluate for thrombosis of the pelvic veins, which may be caused by May-Thurner syndrome (iliac vein thrombosis caused by compression of the left common iliac vein, by the right common iliac artery).[15] Migraine associated with paradoxical embolism via PFO (more common in young patients) is thought caused by a presumed loss of filtration of microemboli or toxic substances via right-to-left shunting.[27,28]

The advantage that TEE possesses relative to TTE is that the US probe is placed in the esophagus and positioned directly behind the heart. This permits the use of higher frequencies because the US beam has a shorter distance to travel. This higher frequency allows a better resolution of images. TEE may have an advantage over TTE in evaluating for bacterial endocarditis, the functioning of prosthetic heart valves, and severe mitral regurgitation caused by ruptured chordae tendineae.

TEE identifies potential causal sources of embolus in patients with CS that leads to changes in management and outcomes at least 3% of the time. Other findings, particularly aorta atherosclerosis, are identified much more commonly but the causal link to stroke is uncertain, thus changes in management in these cases is variable and data describing resulting outcomes are lacking.[29] The utility of TEE and its superiority with respect to TTE is still the subject of discussion.[30]

## Other Diagnostic Modalities

Carotid duplex monitoring for microembolism can detect high-risk patients with asymptomatic carotid stenosis, and assist in identifying mild degrees of symptomatic carotid stenosis in patients with CS. Recently, three-dimensional US and contrast-enhanced US have been used to assess vulnerable plaque at risk for rupture in patients with carotid atherosclerotic disease.[31,32]

In ICU management of cerebrovascular disease, transcranial Doppler (TCD) has typically been used to detect vasospasm after subarachnoid hemorrhage (SAH).[33] It has also been a reliable tool in detecting occlusions of the main intracranial vessels, such as the middle cerebral artery (MCA), or the basilar artery (BA). As the emergency treatment of acute IS evolves, TCD can play an important role because it rapidly, non-invasively, and objectively identifies patients with occlusion of major intracranial arteries who could be candidates for thrombolytic treatment. In addition, it is a reliable tool for the detection of spontaneous or medically induced reperfusion in a previously occluded vessel.[34,35]

Agitated saline TCD monitoring is based on intracranial detection of IV injected microemboli. The size and functional relevance of right-to-left shunting is readily assessed using TCD, with similar sensitivity and specificity with TEE.[35] The reasons that TCD is more sensitive than TEE for detecting PFO, includes the ability to perform a more vigorous Valsalva maneuver in the absence of sedation and the loud and obvious signal that is produced by bubbles on TCD.[34]

## LABORATORY WORK-UP

- Serum lab testing can take on a life of it's own. Basic serum testing would include; glucose, HbA1c, electrolytes, renal function tests, CBC including platelet count, prothrombin time (PT), international normalized ration (INR), activated partial thromboplastin time (aPTT), and HCG for women of child bearing age.
- Other labs to consider; lipid profile, LFTs, TSH with reflex, CRP, ESR, Troponin and CK.
- C-reacdtive protein (CRP), a biomarker for inflammation: elevated level in patients with AFib compared with those who do not have AFib history; patients with persistent AFib have higher CRP levels than those with paroxysmal AFib.[36]
- Brain natriuretic peptide (BNP): assessing cardiac stretch and heart failure, may harbor an underlying or occult cardioembolic mechanism
- Troponin: early positive troponin after IS may be independently associated with a cardiac embolic source
- D dimer: acutely elevated after stroke suggests embolic phenomenon; may implicate a hypercoagulable state due to an occult malignancy
- Fibrinogen (factor I): protein essential for blood clot formation
- Thyroid stimulating hormone (TSH): hyper thyroid can be related to AFib, hypo thyroid can be related to progression of athero
- Homocysteine: amino acid produced as the body digests protein
- Lipoprotein (a): molecule of "bad" cholesterol with an extra protein attached; interferes with blood's natural clot busters
- Venereal disease research laboratory (VDRL): screen for syphilis.

## HYPERCOAGULABLE PROFILE

Evaluating for a hypercoagulable state includes antiphospholipid antibodies (anticardiolipin antibodies, lupus anticoagulant, $\beta_2$ glycoprotein antibody) and genetic mutations (protein C or S deficiency, antithrombin III deficiency, factor V Leiden, prothrombin gene mutation). Of these, only the antiphospholipid antibodies are associated with arterial and venous thromboembolism, and so could potentially cause a stroke if a PFO or other shunt between the venous and arterial circulation is present.[15]

Serum testing for acquired antiphospholipid syndrome may be considered in the presence of a history of prior venous thromboembolism, second trimester abortion, or rheumatologic disorder. The diagnosis requires the persistence of high titers of autoantibodies of the IgG or IgM isotype (for >12 weeks), detected by enzyme-linked immunosorbent assay for anti-β2-glycoprotein I or anticardiolipin antibodies or by lupus-anticoagulant assays.

Other conditions associated with an acquired hypercoagulable state include pregnancy, hormonal contraceptive use, exposure to hormonal treatments (eg, anabolic steroids or erythropoietin), nephritic syndrome, and cancer. Patients with cancer may have distinctive D dimer levels (a marker of coagulopathy, >20 times higher than those without cancer) and infarct patterns (multiple lesions in multiple vascular territories).[37]

IS may be caused by inherited thrombophilia. Tests for thrombophilia have high costs and low diagnostic accuracy. Their results can fluctuate, and repeated assessment is needed or genetic testing should be done where possible. Clues for a hypercoagulable state include a history of DVT or multiple miscarriages.[38]

Inherited or acquired hypercoagulopathies are not a well-studied cause for IS and thought to only contribute to a small proportion of IS. Generally, hypercoagulable work-up for antiphospholipid syndrome and coagulopathies is indicated in select patients, particularly those who are young, with a PFO and possibly at risk of paradoxical embolism, with history of unprovoked venous thromboembolism.[39] To contrast, some recent reports suggest there is little benefit to advanced testing for hypercoagulable states in CS, even in young patients and those with PFOs.[40] Furthermore, identification of hypercoagulable patients may not yield risk reduction in recurrent stroke despite therapy.[41] As a result, many clinicians argue that thrombophilia work-up in stroke is an unjustified cost that can lead to unnecessary anticoagulation.[40] Furthermore, in the setting of an acute stroke, some markers of hypercoagulability are transiently or falsely elevated, and the tests may need to be repeated. Therefore, it is often more cost-effective to perform hypercoagulability testing after other tests have been performed, perhaps in the outpatient rather than the hospital setting. (**Box 2**).

---

**Box 2**
**Hypercoagulable testing considerations**

Antiphospholipid antibodies (APLA) are acquired and associated with both arterial and venous thromboembolism.

- Antiphospholipid antibodies (Anticardiolipin antibodies)
- Lupus anticoagulant
- Beta-2 glycoprotein antibody
    Repeat confirmatory testing needed in 6 months due to false positives.

Genetic mutations (abnormal upfront [may be inherited])

- Not Commonly Associated with Stroke
  - Protein C or S deficiency
  - Antithrombin III deficiency
  - Factor V Leiden mutation
  - Prothrombin gene mutation

Primarily associated with venous thromboembolism, could only potentially cause a stroke if a PFO or other shunt between the venous and arterial circulation if present.

---

## EVALUATION FOR MALIGNANCY

Two of the most common causes of death among the elderly are cancers and IS and the associations between them have been described.[37,42,43] The frequency of stroke in patients with cancer is nearly 7%,[44] most of which develop in the first few months after a cancer diagnosis. This is most likely related to hypercoagulability through alterations of the homeostatic cascade, the integrity of the endothelium, and platelet function.[45–47] Stroke mechanisms in patients with known cancer may differ from those that occur in the general population,[42,48] with CS subtype being the most common and associated with reduced survival.[49]

Because of advances in cancer medicine and the growing elderly population, the number of people living with cancer is increasing. As a consequence, the number of patients who have cancer is expected to increase among patients with stroke, especially in those without other stroke pathologic processes. Certain cancers, such as lung cancer (especially adenocarcinoma), and gastrointestinal malignancies secrete substances, such as cysteine proteases, tissue factor, and sialic acid moieties of mucin, and exhibit procoagulant activity, resulting in the activation of factors X and VII.[50,51] Aggressive antitumor therapy may increase the risk of thrombosis.[52] Anticoagulation can effectively prevent cancer-related stroke; hence, early identification of this stroke mechanism is important and requires additional studies.

Once other potential stroke mechanisms are excluded, an evaluation for occult malignancy as a cause of CS should be considered, especially in older patients with systemic symptoms suggestive of a cancer diagnosis, such as unexplained weight loss. Cerebral infarcts involving multiple vascular territories are more common in patients with cancer.[53] There should be a low threshold of diagnostic testing when looking for an occult malignancy in the absence of systemic symptoms suggestive of cancer. Additional testing commonly performed includes age-appropriate cancer screening modalities; serum inflammatory markers, such as erythrocyte sedimentation rate (ESR); and CT scan of the chest, abdomen, and pelvis.[42]

## GENETIC CONSIDERATIONS FOR CRYPTOGENIC STROKE

This topic cannot be adequately addressed in this article. The following is a brief overview of considerations.

Hereditary factors contribute to stroke risk, although teasing apart risk because of genetic mutations and because of shared familial exposures remains challenging. The task has been complicated by the heterogeneity of stroke, the multitude of conventional risk factors that cause stroke, and the variability among populations and studies.[54]

Genetic variability may however, contribute to stroke risk through several potential mechanisms. First, specific rare single-gene disorders may contribute to individual familial syndromes for which stroke is the primary or unique manifestation (eg, cerebral autosomal-dominant arteriopathy with subcortical infarcts and leukoencephalopathy). Second, single-gene disorders may cause a multisystem disorder of which stroke is just one manifestation (eg, sickle cell anemia). Third, some common variants of genetic polymorphisms have been associated with stroke risk, although the individual contribution of such polymorphisms is regarded as modest (eg, variants in 9p21).[55] Fourth, genetic causes of conventional stroke risk factors, such as AFib, diabetes mellitus, and hypertension, are also associated with risk of stroke.[56] Emerging evidence suggests that genetic studies could help to distinguish stroke subtypes and even contribute to patient management. For example, there is an association between gene variations that confer an increased risk of AFib and IS. This raises the possibility that genetic tests could help to make the diagnosis of strokes likely to be because of AFib.[55]

| Genetic causes related to stroke |
| --- |
| • CADASIL - Cerebral autosomal-dominant arteriopathy with subcortical infarcts and leukoencephalopathy |
| • MELAS - Mitochondrial encephalomyopathy lactic acidosis and stroke-like episodes |
| • MTHFR - Methylenetetrahydrofolate reductase |
| • FHM - Familial hemiplegic migraine |
| • APLA - Antiphospholipid antibody |
| • Moyamoya disease (abnormal net-like blood vessels) |
| • Ehlers-Danlos syndrome (connective tissue disorders) |
| • Fabry disease (enzyme alpha-galactosidase A. deficiency) |

## SUBSTANCE USE AND ABUSE

Substance abuse, notably cocaine abuse, is an important risk factor in stroke. In a large population-based study, cocaine use was associated with a 5.7-fold increase in the odds of having an IS in young adults.[57] Furthermore, de los Ríos and colleagues[58] recognized an increased frequency of cocaine abuse as a cause of stroke among 35- to 54-year-old patients with stroke. These observations generate a strong case for aggressive community-based education regarding increasing cocaine abuse and risk for stroke.

Illicit drug use has been associated with increased stroke risk. Cocaine, amphetamines, and heroin substantially increase the risk of hemorrhagic stroke and IS. Adjusting for other risk factors, there is a 7- to 14-fold increase in stroke among drug abusers. Pathogenesis is likely multifactorial. Hypertension, vasospasm, intravascular thrombosis caused by platelet activation and vasculitis. Cocaine functions by blocking the presynaptic reuptake of dopamine, norepinephrine, and serotonin. Elevated levels of these monoamines have been angiographically proven to cause cerebral artery vasoconstriction.[59–61]

In one of the earliest studies looking at the cardiovascular effects manifested by cannabis, Mittleman and colleagues[62] reported a nearly five-fold increased risk of myocardial infarction (MI) within an hour of consuming cannabis. Several mechanisms by which cannabis negatively impacts the cardiovascular system has been hypothesized in case reports.[63] These include orthostatic hypotension, cardiac arrhythmias, and intimal hyperplasia (response of a vessel to injury). In addition, a prospective study of 48 young patients with IS demonstrated a strong temporal association of cannabis consumption and reversible cerebral vasoconstriction syndrome (RCVS).[64] An Australian cohort of young patients with stroke revealed that cannabis users had a 2.3-fold higher risk for developing IS even when adjusted for all other covariates including tobacco use.[65]

Similarly, a population-based study used the US nationwide inpatient sample and demonstrated that smoking cannabis was independently associated with the occurrence of stroke. The mean age at stroke was 33.1 years.[66] In contrast, a Swedish study failed to identify this independent relationship among young adults.[64] With the societal drift for increased cannabis legalization for medical and recreational use, its use may not be as harmless as otherwise thought of, and more research is needed to explore the potential relationship between cannabis use and stroke.

## INFECTIOUS CONSIDERATIONS

The association of stroke with infectious entities, such as infectious endocarditis, has been well described,[67] but direct infectious causes outside the realm of infectious endocarditis continues to be an area of debate. This becomes more relevant in strokes deemed as cryptogenic or of undetermined cause.[68]

Consider lumbar puncture (LP) to look for signs of an infectious, inflammatory, or neoplastic valvular lesion; atrial clot; or aortic atherosclerosis. In certain clinical settings, such as immunosuppressed patients or those with high exposure risk, and in patients with evidence of multifocal infarcts, infectious etiologies, such as viruses (varicella-zoster virus, herpes simplex virus, and cytomegalovirus), syphilis, and tuberculosis, should be considered and confirmed by serum and cerebrospinal fluid (CSF) testing.[14] Obtain blood cultures if there is concern for infectious endocarditis. Procalcitonin and BioFire testing may be prudent to consider.

Infections increase the susceptibility to stroke by causing local inflammation of the cerebral parenchyma and meninges, through systemic inflammation, by promoting atherosclerosis, causing coagulation and endothelial dysfunction, and in some cases directly inducing ischemia.[69,70] Another proposed mechanism describes a direct pathogenic invasion of the vascular wall with smooth muscle cell proliferation or increased cytokine production, or a combination of both.[71] Inflammation seems to be a common pathway in stroke causation with infection. Persistent inflammatory activity even after a resolved infection has been shown to increase stroke risk years later.[72]

Infectious causes of stroke are underrecognized, but are important to consider in pediatric patients, young adults with no apparent vascular risk factors, immunocompromised patients, and in patients with cryptogenic ischemic or hemorrhagic stroke. Inflammation in the setting of infection seems to increase the risk of cerebrovascular events. Identifying infectious causes is challenging, hence a high index of suspicion and a low threshold for obtaining additional nontraditional stroke investigations is necessary, especially in the aforementioned high-risk patients. These investigations can include contrast cerebral imaging, cerebrospinal fluid analysis, and high-resolution vessel imaging modalities that may facilitate an early diagnosis and prompt initiation of targeted antimicrobial therapy.[73]

Preventive and therapeutic interventions through the use of vaccinations and antibiotic therapy along with having a low threshold for infectious evaluation in select patients may, help in reducing the stroke incidence.[73]

## SUMMARY

The specific cause of stroke in a large number of patients continues to challenge clinicians despite efforts to arrive at a CS diagnosis. Approximately 30% to 40% of ischemic strokes do not have a definitive cause despite specialized, costly testing, that often results in diminishing yield. Understanding the pathogenic mechanism of stroke, lack of Class I evidence, the workup and treatment strategies often vary considerably. CS incorporates a heterogenous group of patients leading to therapeutic implications based on the potential mechanism. In the absence of AFib, antiplatelet therapy continues to be the mainstay of treatment, though scientific evidence to support this is limited. In addition, risk factor management and lifestyle modifications, lead to improved stroke prevention strategies in patients with CS.

## DISCLOSURE

The author has nothing to disclose.

## REFERENCES

1. Bogousslavsky J, Caplan LR. Uncommon causes of stroke. Cambridge: Cambridge University Press; 2001.
2. Sacco RL, Ellenberg J, Mohr J, et al. Infarcts of undetermined cause: the NINCDS stroke data bank. Ann Neurol 1989;25(4):382–90.
3. Hart RG, Halperin JL. Atrial fibrillation and stroke: concepts and controversies. Stroke 2001;32(3):803–8.
4. Ryan D. Handbook of neuroscience nursing: care of the adult neurosurgical patient. New York: Thieme; 2019.
5. Adams HP, Bendixen BH, Kappelle LJ, et al. Classification of subtype of acute ischemic stroke. definitions for use in a multicenter clinical trial. TOAST. trial of org 10172 in acute stroke treatment. Stroke 1993;24(1):35–41.
6. Etherton MR, Rost NS, Wu O. Infarct topography and functional outcomes. J Cereb Blood Flow Metab 2018;38(9):1517–32.
7. Liberman AL, Prabhakaran S. Cryptogenic stroke: how to define it? how to treat it? Curr Cardiol Rep 2013;15(12):423.
8. Hart RG, Diener H, Coutts SB, et al. Embolic strokes of undetermined source: the case for a new clinical construct. Lancet Neurol 2014;13(4):429–38.
9. O'Donnell M, Kasner SE. Cryptogenic stroke. In: Grotta J, Albers G, Broderick J, et al, editors. Stroke. 6th edition. New York: Elsevier; 2016. p. 707–15.
10. Hart RG, Catanese L, Perera KS, et al. Embolic stroke of undetermined source: a systematic review and clinical update. Stroke 2017;48(4):867–72.
11. Saver JL. Cryptogenic stroke. N Engl J Med 2016;374(21):2065–74.
12. Goldstein LB, Bushnell CD, Adams RJ, et al. Guidelines for the primary prevention of stroke: a guideline for healthcare professionals from the American Heart Association/American Stroke Association. Stroke 2011;42(2):517–84.
13. Ovbiagele B, Goldstein LB, Higashida RT, et al. Forecasting the future of stroke in the United States: a policy statement from the American Heart Association and American Stroke Association. Stroke 2013;44(8):2361–75.
14. Yaghi S, Elkind MS. Cryptogenic stroke: a diagnostic challenge. Neurol Clin Pract 2014;4(5):386–93.
15. Berkowitz A. Lange clinical neurology and neuroanatomy: a localization-based approach. New York: McGraw-Hill Education; 2016.
16. Kelley RE, Kovacs AG. Mechanism of in-hospital cerebral ischemia. Stroke 1986;17(3):430–3.
17. Azzimondi G, Nonino F, Fiorani L, et al. Incidence of stroke among inpatients in a large Italian hospital. Stroke 1994;25(9):1752–4.
18. Singh V, Edwards NJ. Advances in the critical care management of ischemic stroke. Stroke Res Treat 2013;2013:510481.
19. Rubens JR, Selvaggio G, Lu TK. Synthetic mixed-signal computation in living cells. Nat Commun 2016;7:11658.
20. Powers WJ, Rabinstein AA, Ackerson T, et al. 2018 guidelines for the early management of patients with acute ischemic stroke: a guideline for healthcare professionals from the American Heart Association/American Stroke Association. Stroke 2018;49(3):e46–99.
21. Chalela JA, Kidwell CS, Nentwich LM, et al. Magnetic resonance imaging and computed tomography in emergency assessment of patients with suspected acute stroke: a prospective comparison. Lancet 2007;369(9558):293–8.
22. Merino JG, Warach S. Imaging of acute stroke. Nat Rev Neurol 2010;6(10):560.

23. Liao J, Khalid Z, Scallan C, et al. Noninvasive cardiac monitoring for detecting paroxysmal atrial fibrillation or flutter after acute ischemic stroke: a systematic review. Stroke 2007;38(11):2935–40.

24. Connolly SJ, Eikelboom J, Joyner C, et al. Apixaban in patients with atrial fibrillation. N Engl J Med 2011;364(9):806–17.

25. Sanna T, Diener H, Passman RS, et al. Cryptogenic stroke and underlying atrial fibrillation. N Engl J Med 2014;370(26):2478–86.

26. Choe WC, Passman RS, Brachmann J, et al. A comparison of atrial fibrillation monitoring strategies after cryptogenic stroke (from the cryptogenic stroke and underlying AF trial). Am J Cardiol 2015;116(6):889–93.

27. Diener H, Weimar C, Katsarava Z. Patent foramen ovale: paradoxical connection to migraine and stroke. Curr Opin Neurol 2005;18(3):299–304.

28. Dao CN, Tobis JM. PFO and paradoxical embolism producing events other than stroke. Catheter Cardiovasc Interv 2011;77(6):903–9.

29. Christiansen ME, Van Woerkom RC, Demaerschalk BM, et al. What is clinical efficacy of transesophageal echocardiography in patients with cryptogenic stroke? A critically appraised topic. Neurologist 2018;23(1):30–3.

30. de Bruijn SF, Agema WR, Lammers GJ, et al. Transesophageal echocardiography is superior to transthoracic echocardiography in management of patients of any age with transient ischemic attack or stroke. Stroke 2006;37(10):2531–4.

31. Madani A, Beletsky V, Tamayo A, et al. High-risk asymptomatic carotid stenosis: ulceration on 3D ultrasound vs TCD microemboli. Neurology 2011;77(8):744–50.

32. Partovi S, Loebe M, Aschwanden M, et al. Contrast-enhanced ultrasound for assessing carotid atherosclerotic plaque lesions. Am J Roentgenol 2012;198(1): W13–9.

33. Sloan MA, Alexandrov AV, Tegeler CH, et al. Assessment: transcranial Doppler ultrasonography: report of the therapeutics and technology assessment subcommittee of the American Academy of Neurology. Neurology 2004;62(9):1468–81.

34. Kulkarni AA, Sharma VK. Role of transcranial Doppler in cerebrovascular disease. Neurol India 2016;64(5):995–1001.

35. Mitsias P. Ischemic stroke management in the critical care unit: the first 24 hours. J Stroke Cerebrovasc Dis 1999;8(3):151–9.

36. Chung MK, Martin DO, Sprecher D, et al. C-reactive protein elevation in patients with atrial arrhythmias: inflammatory mechanisms and persistence of atrial fibrillation. Circulation 2001;104(24):2886–91.

37. Kim SJ, Park JH, Lee M, et al. Clues to occult cancer in patients with ischemic stroke. PLoS One 2012;7(9):e44959.

38. Berlit P. Diagnosis and treatment of cerebral vasculitis. Ther Adv Neurol Disord 2010;3(1):29–42.

39. Reynolds HR, Jagen MA, Tunick PA, et al. Sensitivity of transthoracic versus transesophageal echocardiography for the detection of native valve vegetations in the modern era. J Am Soc Echocardiogr 2003;16(1):67–70.

40. Morris JG, Singh S, Fisher M. Testing for inherited thrombophilias in arterial stroke: can it cause more harm than good? Stroke 2010;41(12):2985–90.

41. Kolominsky-Rabas PL, Weber M, Gefeller O, et al. Epidemiology of ischemic stroke subtypes according to TOAST criteria: incidence, recurrence, and long-term survival in ischemic stroke subtypes: a population-based study. Stroke 2001;32(12):2735–40.

42. Seok JM, Kim SG, Kim JW, et al. Coagulopathy and embolic signal in cancer patients with ischemic stroke. Ann Neurol 2010;68(2):213–9.

43. Kim SG, Hong JM, Kim HY, et al. Ischemic stroke in cancer patients with and without conventional mechanisms: a multicenter study in Korea. Stroke 2010; 41(4):798–801.

44. Graus F, Rogers LR, Posner JB. Cerebrovascular complications in patients with cancer. Medicine (Baltimore) 1985;64(1):16–35.

45. Caine GJ, Stonelake PS, Lip GY, et al. The hypercoagulable state of malignancy: pathogenesis and current debate. Neoplasia 2002;4(6):465–73.

46. Dammacco F, Vacca A, Procaccio P, et al. Cancer-related coagulopathy (trousseau's syndrome): review of the literature and experience of a single center of internal medicine. Clin Exp Med 2013;13(2):85–97.

47. Sack GH, Levin J, Bell WR. Trousseau's syndrome and other manifestations of chronic disseminated coagulopathy in patients with neoplasms: clinical, pathophysiologic, and therapeutic features. Medicine (Baltimore) 1977;56(1):1–37.

48. Schwarzbach CJ, Schaefer A, Ebert A, et al. Stroke and cancer: the importance of cancer-associated hypercoagulation as a possible stroke etiology. Stroke 2012;43(11):3029–34.

49. Navi BB, Singer S, Merkler AE, et al. Recurrent thromboembolic events after ischemic stroke in patients with cancer. Neurology 2014;83(1):26–33.

50. Bick RL. Cancer-associated thrombosis. N Engl J Med 2003;349(2):109–11.

51. Rickles FR, Patierno S, Fernandez PM. Tissue factor, thrombin, and cancer. Chest 2003;124(3):58S–68S.

52. Li S, Chen W, Tang Y, et al. Incidence of ischemic stroke post-chemotherapy: a retrospective review of 10,963 patients. Clin Neurol Neurosurg 2006;108(2):150–6.

53. Giray S, Sarica FB, Arlier Z, et al. Recurrent ischemic stroke as an initial manifestation of an concealed pancreatic adenocarcinoma: Trousseau's syndrome. Chin Med J 2011;124(4):637–40.

54. Boehme AK, Esenwa C, Elkind MS. Stroke risk factors, genetics, and prevention. Circ Res 2017;120(3):472–95.

55. Gretarsdottir S, Thorleifsson G, Manolescu A, et al. Risk variants for atrial fibrillation on chromosome 4q25 associate with ischemic stroke. Ann Neurol 2008;64(4): 402–9.

56. Bevan S, Traylor M, Adib-Samii P, et al. Genetic heritability of ischemic stroke and the contribution of previously reported candidate gene and genomewide associations. Stroke 2012;43(12):3161–7.

57. Cheng Y, Ryan KA, Qadwai SA, et al. Cocaine use and risk of ischemic stroke in young adults. Stroke 2016;47(4):918–22.

58. de los Ríos F, Kleindorfer DO, Khoury J, et al. Trends in substance abuse preceding stroke among young adults: a population-based study. Stroke 2012;43(12): 3179–83.

59. Amin H, Greer DM. Cryptogenic stroke: the appropriate diagnostic evaluation. Curr Treat Options Cardiovasc Med 2014;16(1):280.

60. Ionita CC, Xavier AR, Kirmani JF, et al. What proportion of stroke is not explained by classic risk factors? Prev Cardiol 2005;8(1):41–6.

61. Kaufman MJ, Levin JM, Ross MH, et al. Cocaine-induced cerebral vasoconstriction detected in humans with magnetic resonance angiography. JAMA 1998; 279(5):376–80.

62. Mittleman MA, Lewis RA, Maclure M, et al. Triggering myocardial infarction by marijuana. Circulation 2001;103(23):2805–9.

63. Wolff V, Armspach J, Lauer V, et al. Cannabis-related stroke: myth or reality? Stroke 2013;44(2):558–63.

64. Falkstedt D, Wolff V, Allebeck P, et al. Cannabis, tobacco, alcohol use, and the risk of early stroke: a population-based cohort study of 45 000 Swedish men. Stroke 2017;48(2):265–70.
65. Hemachandra D, McKetin R, Cherbuin N, et al. Heavy cannabis users at elevated risk of stroke: evidence from a general population survey. Aust N Z J Public Health 2016;40(3):226–30.
66. Kalla A, Krishnamoorthy PM, Gopalakrishnan A, et al. Cannabis use predicts risks of heart failure and cerebrovascular accidents: results from the national inpatient sample. J Cardiovasc Med 2018;19(9):480–4.
67. Silver B, Behrouz R, Silliman S. Bacterial endocarditis and cerebrovascular disease. Curr Neurol Neurosci Rep 2016;16(12):104.
68. Yaghi S, Bernstein RA, Passman R, et al. Cryptogenic stroke: research and practice. Circ Res 2017;120(3):527–40.
69. Manousakis G, Jensen MB, Chacon MR, et al. The interface between stroke and infectious disease: infectious diseases leading to stroke and infections complicating stroke. Curr Neurol Neurosci Rep 2009;9(1):28.
70. Bergh C, Fall K, Udumyan R, et al. Severe infections and subsequent delayed cardiovascular disease. Eur J Prev Cardiol 2017;24(18):1958–66.
71. Fugate JE, Lyons JL, Thakur KT, et al. Infectious causes of stroke. Lancet Infect Dis 2014;14(9):869–80.
72. Ihara M, Yamamoto Y. Emerging evidence for pathogenesis of sporadic cerebral small vessel disease. Stroke 2016;47(2):554–60.
73. Jillella DV, Wisco DR. Infectious causes of stroke. Curr Opin Infect Dis 2019;32(3):285–92.

# Management of the Patient with Malignant Hemispheric Stroke

Mary McKenna Guanci, MSN, RN, CNRN, SCRN

## KEYWORDS

- Malignant middle cerebral artery stroke • Decompressive hemicraniectomy
- Cerebral edema • Herniation

## KEY POINTS

- MMCA stroke has a high mortality and morbidity rate despite aggressive intervention.
- Patients may present with cerebral edema or have a high risk to develop edema within 3 to 72 hours.
- Decompressive hemicraniectomy (DHC) is a lifesaving surgery, but may not be beneficial in improving functional outcome especially in those patients greater than 60 years of age.
- Nurses have an important role in shepherding the patient and family through the uncertain hospital course and advocating for care decisions that would be acceptable to the patient.

## INTRODUCTION

A malignant hemispheric stroke, also known as a malignant middle cerebral artery (MMCA) stroke, is a term used to describe a thromboembolic stroke that occurs in the entire middle cerebral artery (MCA) trunk or in the distal internal carotid artery resulting in space-occupying cerebral edema that occurs immediately or within a period of 5 days.[1] MMCA stroke occurs in 10% of all ischemic strokes but has a much higher patient mortality rate attributed to the increased risk of cerebral edema and herniation. Impaired consciousness can develop 3 hours after symptom onset and progress to death with a mortality rate estimated to be 70% to 80% despite intervention and aggressive intensive care.[2] A collaborative interdisciplinary team approach is needed to manage these complex stroke patients. The nurse plays a vital role in bedside management, not only in clinical assessment and intervention, but in support of the patient and family through this complex course of care.

## PATHOPHYSIOLOGY

The MCA territory is divided into the superior, inferior, and lenticulostriate arteries. The MCAs rise from the internal carotid artery and supply most of the lateral surface of the

Massachusetts General Hospital, Lunder Building 6th Floor ICU, 55 Fruit St, Boston, MA 02114, USA
E-mail address: jmtkac@comcast.net

Crit Care Nurs Clin N Am 32 (2020) 51–66
https://doi.org/10.1016/j.cnc.2019.11.003
0899-5885/20/© 2019 Elsevier Inc. All rights reserved.
ccnursing.theclinics.com

cerebral hemispheres, except for the superior portion of the parietal lobes and the inferior portion of the temporal and occipital lobes. It is also responsible for blood flow to the internal capsule and basal ganglia (**Fig. 1**).

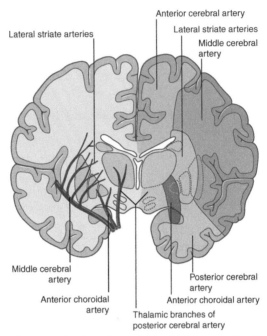

**Fig. 1.** Distribution of perforating branches of the middle cerebral, anterior choroidal, and posterior cerebral arteries (schematic). The anterior choroidal artery arises from the internal carotid. (*From* Mtui E, Gruener G, Dockery P. Blood supply of the brain. In: Fitzgerald's clinical neuroanatomy and neuroscience. 7th edition. Philadelphia: Elsevier; 2016. p. 53; with permission.)

## MALIGNANT CEREBRAL EDEMA

There is no known mortality difference between right versus left hemispheric strokes; however, there may be a higher incidence of malignant transformation in those patients with right hemispheric MMCA stroke. A thromboembolic event of the MCA produces an inflammatory cascade that often results in cytotoxic (cell swelling caused by intracellular accumulation of fluid) and vasogenic edema (extracellular accumulation of fluid resulting from disruption of the blood-brain barrier [BBB]). Rastogi and colleagues[3] described the insula region of each hemisphere as playing a role in the regulation of the autonomic nervous system (ANS), and greater alterations of the ANS are seen in right versus left insular strokes. This may lead to higher mortality for right insular strokes versus left at 3 months.[4] The edema formation following the ischemic event may be described as follows:

- A thromboembolic stroke of the MCA produces ANS dysregulation and release of norepinephrine leading to ischemic damage.
- Norepinephrine release stimulates the hypothalamic-pituitary access.
- The hypothalamic-pituitary access regulates vasopressin release. Vasopressin release induces the downregulation of aquaporin 4, increasing

plasma membrane permeability and increased edema through inflammatory pathways.
- ANS dysregulation results in increased glutamate release and vasoconstriction leading to calcium increases, sodium and potassium pump failure, and osmotic changes to the BBB and results in cerebral edema (**Fig. 2**).

Other mechanisms that contribute to MMCA edema and secondary injury are being investigated including the role of cortical spreading depolarization or depression. Cortical spreading depression represents a wave of depolarization in the gray matter as seen on electroencephalogram (EEG); this depolarization may contribute to the alteration of the BBB, leading to edema. Episodes of cortical spreading depression have been recorded on EEG in many MMCA patients.[5] Future studies of cortical spreading depression impact on ischemia in MMCA stroke may influence intensive care unit (ICU) interventions, such as blood pressure (BP) management, fever prevention, and oxygenation that may further better patient outcomes.

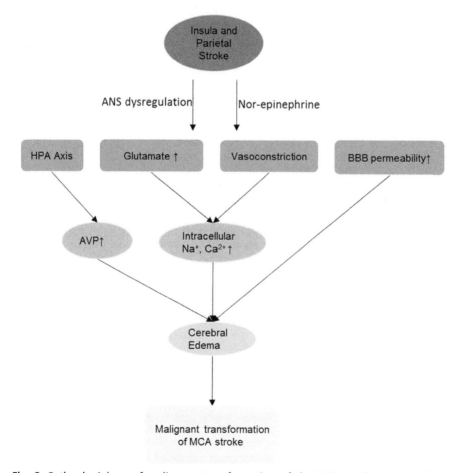

**Fig. 2.** Pathophysiology of malignant transformation of the MCA stroke. AVP, arginine vasopressin; HPA, hypothalamic-pituitary axis. (*From* Rastogi V, Lamb DG, Williamson JB. Hemispheric differences in malignant middle cerebral artery stroke. J Neurol Sci. 2015;353(1–2):25; with permission.)

## PREDICTING AT-RISK PATIENTS

Patients with MMCA stroke typically present with signs of herniation on admission. Those at risk for developing malignant hemispheric cerebral edema often exhibit a decreasing level of consciousness (LOC), pupillary changes, motor weakness, and respiratory deterioration. It is estimated that one-third of MMCA stroke patients deteriorate within 24 hours.[2] Early prediction of patients at risk to deteriorate would assist the clinical team with decision-making regarding the clinical interventions that may be required including hyperosmolar therapy and decompressive hemicraniectomy (DHC). More importantly, early prediction may inform neuroprognostication assisting the team and family who are often acting as surrogate decision makers.

Clinical studies have concentrated on exploring radiographic and biomarker predictors, but to date there is no single predictor that can be relied on. Computed tomography (CT) is used in the early evaluation. This is especially helpful in facilities where MRI is limited or unavailable. CT following stroke demonstrates hypoattenuation in the white matter. If these areas exceed 50% of the MCA territory, malignant infarction is predicted to occur. Infarct volume greater than 22 mL and a midline shift of greater than 3.9 mm predicts severe edema and herniation.[6] The use of CT-perfusion studies aids in examining the BBB and permeability, and also helps to predict edema formation. Perfusion studies and CT angiography assist in assessing cerebral blood vessels, vascular territories, and collateral circulation (**Fig. 3**). The Alberta Stroke Program Early CT Score (ASPECTS score) is a 10-point (CT) scoring system used to measure infarcted tissue and cytotoxic edema following stroke. The CT is examined in 10 specific target areas of the MCA, basal ganglia, and supraganglionic areas. Ten is the highest possible score and represents a low risk for ischemic change. A score of −1 is subtracted from 10 for each area of ischemia found in the target area (**Fig. 4**). An ASPECTS score less than or equal to seven predicts the development of cerebral edema.[7] More recently, the ASPECTS score has been used in clinical decision making regarding the benefit of endovascular thrombectomy (EVT) in patients with MMCA stroke. Patients with a low ASPECTS score demonstrate decreased edema formation following successful recanalization.[8] MRI using diffusion-weighted imaging sequences also provides early detection of ischemic changes. Diffusion-weighted imaging measures lesion volume, which if greater than 145 mL is predictive of a malignant infarction.[6]

A combined early prediction approach using radiographic and clinical parameters is suggested for early identification of those patients who are at risk. A National Institute of Health stroke scale (NIHSS) greater than 10, patient characteristics that include young age (<78 years), hypoattenuation on CT greater than 50% of MCA territory at 6 to 40 hours, and MRI with diffusion-weighted image greater than 82 mL at 6 hours or greater than 145 mL at 14 hours have been described as helpful predictors.[9,10]

## ADMISSION PATHWAY

The patient with an MMCA stroke presents to the emergency department and is managed on the acute stroke response pathway. These patients are at an increased risk of hemispheric injury causing a decreased LOC resulting in airway compromise and intubation. Treatment decisions including the use of alteplase or EVT are based on time last known well, physical examination quantified by the NIHSS, vital signs, and CT results. When the diagnosis of MMCA stroke is suspected, consulting neurosurgery is essential to consider the risk/benefit for decompressive craniotomy. Triage to another facility should be expedited if neurosurgical services or a dedicated neuroscience ICU are not available because of the high risk for neurologic deterioration.[9]

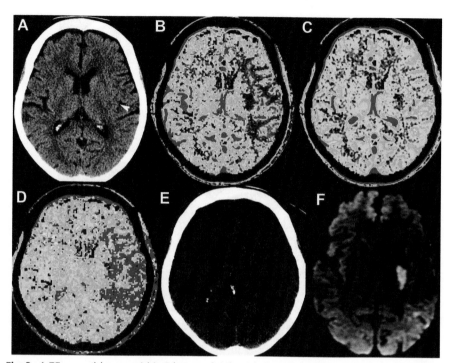

**Fig. 3.** A 75-year-old man, within 2 hours of right-sided stroke and presentation of NIHSS 20. (A) Non-contrast CT (NCCT) demonstrates subtle loss of the left posterior putamen, internal capsule, and posterior insular cortex (*white arrowhead*) (ASPECTS 7). (B) Cerebral blood flow. (C) Cerebral blood volume. (D) Mean transit time. Cerebral blood volume demonstrates an abnormality confined to the posterior putamen and internal capsule (ASPECTS 8), with larger cerebral blood flow and mean transit-time abnormalities corresponding to the left middle cerebral artery M1 segment occlusion (not shown). (E) Follow-up NCCT at Day 6 shows an indistinct posterior putamen confirmed on diffusion-weighted MRI (F). The patient recovered by 18 points with a final NIHSS of 2. NCCT; NIHSS, National Institute of Health stroke scale. (*From* Aviv R, Mandelcorn J, Chakraborty S, et al. Alberta Stroke Program Early CT Scoring of CT perfusion in early stroke visualization and assessment. AJNR Am J Neuroradiol. 2007;28(10):1976; with permission.)

After MMCA stroke is determined, CT ASPECTS score and, if available, MRI are again reviewed for patient eligibility for EVT or emergency DHC. DHC is not contraindicated in patients exhibiting edema related to MMCA stroke.[9,11] The Endovascular Stroke Treatment's Impact on Malignant Type of Edema (ESTIMATE) study evaluated edema formation, mortality rates, and outcomes in MMCA stroke patients. EVT intervention may decrease the risk of MMCA edema development and improve mortality rates and favorable outcomes in these patients at discharge.[12] After the treatment plan is determined, the patient is admitted to a neuroscience ICU.

## PATIENT MANAGEMENT

The patient with MMCA stroke requires the care of a multidisciplinary team with neuroscience expertise. The ideal team consists of an attending physician, fellow, resident, and/or nurse practitioner, nurse, respiratory therapist, and pharmacist who round together at least daily. Physical, occupational, and speech therapy, along with

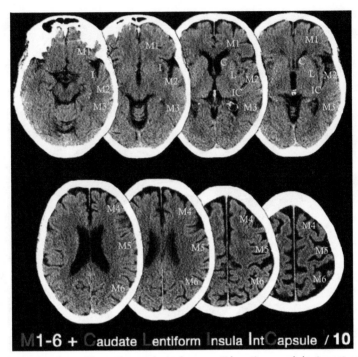

**Fig. 4.** ASPECTS regions. (*From* Aspectsinstroke.com, Education module Aspect and mCTA. Calgary Stroke Program; with permission.)

physiatry, assist with determining functional outcome and an appropriate discharge plan with case management.[13] Social work and chaplaincy aid in support to the patient and family throughout the hospitalization.[14–16] General care decisions for MMCA patients are guided by acute stroke management and ICU guidelines; however, there are some unique neurologic intensive care needs specific to this high-risk patient population that should be considered.

## AIRWAY/RESPIRATORY MANAGEMENT

Patients presenting with MMCA stroke often present with an altered LOC that may require intubation and mechanical ventilation because of the patients' inability to protect their airway.[17] Patient management requires ventilator parameters and weaning strategies, head of bed (HOB) elevation 30°, chest physical therapy, and early mobilization per ICU guidelines.

Hyperventilation can often be used briefly to decrease carbon dioxide ($CO_2$) levels in the emergency management of intubated MMCA stroke patients with increased intracranial pressure (ICP). $CO_2$ is a potent cerebral vasodilator, causing increased cerebral blood volume in an already edematous brain and cranial cavity with minimal space. Reducing $CO_2$ via hyperventilation results in cerebral vasoconstriction, decreased blood volume, and a decrease in ICP. This response, however, is temporary and if hyperventilation is sustained there is a risk of rebound vasodilation and increased infarct volume resulting again in increasing ICP. Hyperventilation is therefore avoided except as a bridge to other treatments during emergency resuscitation.[18,19] Decreased LOC, dysphagia, and cognitive impairments increase the risk for ineffective airway clearance. Keeping HOB elevated at 30°, providing oral care, chest physical therapy, and the completion of a swallow screen before anything by mouth is given are critical to preventing aspiration. If the patient is unable to swallow, and if within goals of care (GOC) a nasogastric or orogastric tube should be placed for enteral feeding and medication access.[20–22] Depending on the severity of the neurologic examination and GOC, tracheostomy and percutaneous gastrostomy placement may be necessary to ensure safety, and minimize risk of complications including aspiration, immobility, infection, and skin breakdown as the patient moves though the care continuum.

## ASSESSMENT

Patients with MMCA stroke may present with ipsilateral (same side as the stroke) gaze preference, contralateral (opposite side) sensorimotor deficits, contralateral neglect, and contralateral visual field deficit. Dominant hemispheric strokes may involve language deficits and in larger strokes like MMCA receptive, expressive, and global aphasia. The dominant hemisphere is usually identified by handedness. The left hemisphere is the dominant hemisphere of a right-handed person; however, this is not the case in people who are left-handed. The left hemisphere is still the dominant hemisphere in 65% of left-handed dominant patients creating uncertainty in predicting outcome for patients who are unable to have language tested.[19]

The MMCA stroke patient not only presents with significant neurologic deficits but has an increased risk for developing clinical signs of hemispheric cerebral herniation. This includes an altered LOC, ipsilateral pupil change evolving to bilateral fixed and dilated pupils, and a decline in purposeful response to pain deteriorating to decerebrate (extension) or decorticate (flexion) posturing. Decerebrate posturing is described as an involuntary rigid extension and inward rotation of the arms and legs and decorticate posturing as involuntary rigid flexion or the arms and extension of the legs when a painful stimulus is applied. These examination changes may alter respiratory rate and pattern, increase BP and decrease heart rate.[18,20,23]

The bedside examination and the use of serial CTs are two significant strategies used to monitor the MMCA stroke patient for increasing cerebral edema. The nurse plays a pivotal role in the detection of any neurologic change.[18] LOC is the most sensitive indicator of increasing cerebral edema and resulting herniation and monitoring for changes is critical. Assessing LOC may be difficult when cognitive and language deficits and motor pathway disturbances impair the ability of the patient to "obey commands" as a test for wakefulness or arousability. An example is eyelid apraxia (eye opening) or the inability of some MMCA stroke patients to open eyes to command because of motor pathway disturbance. This requires the examiner to hold open the patient's eyes to engage the patient in an examination because the patient is unable to do so.[19]

Clinicians should avoid or minimize the use of sedatives and analgesia medications used for patient management that will also interfere with the ability to assess the LOC especially during the peak period of cerebral edema risk, which typically occurs up to 5 days. If sedation is required for agitation or ventilator synchrony, agents chosen should be short acting to allow for LOC examination. Propofol (Diprivan) and dexmedetomidine (Precedex) are two intravenous medications commonly used if sedation is necessary. Diprivan is a short-acting, lipophilic intravenous general anesthetic. It has a short half-life and may be turned off for examination testing and resumed if indicated. It does require the patient be intubated for use and is not recommended in the pediatric population because of risk of propofol infusion syndrome.[23] Dexmedetomidine, is an $\alpha_2$-adrenergic antagonist, has rapid distribution, and does not accumulate, enabling neurologic examinations without discontinuation and may be used in intubated or nonintubated patients.[24] It does inhibit sympathetic activity and may decrease BP and heart rate. When possible, nasogastric or orogastric tube medications are encouraged rather than the more sedating intravenous analgesia, pain, and anxiolytic medications. Assessment of all medication regimes during team rounds is suggested as a best practice strategy to maximize patient comfort and minimize risk of post-ICU syndrome. Post-ICU syndrome is described as a sequela of cognitive, motor, and sensory deficits experienced by the patient months after ICU discharge and believed to be caused by prolonged sedation, ventilation, and immobility experienced during ICU management.[25]

There is no evidence to guide the team in how often a neurologic examination should be completed. Decisions concerning timing of neurologic examination should consider deterioration risk, sleep deprivation, and potential delirium concerns. Given the high risk for neurologic deterioration in the acute phase, best practice dictates considerations of an examination that includes LOC, pupillary size and reactivity, along with motor response every 1 to 2 hours with re-evaluation of these intervals as a patient's risk of edema and cerebral herniation decreases. The use of a pupillary device (pupilometer) to measure size and reactivity can provide quantitative, objective information used to evaluate incremental patient change.[26] Any change in examination findings is reported immediately and an emergency CT is obtained. MRI may also be desirable to assess the volume of edema (water), which may aid in evaluation of edema formation. If traveling to CT scan, best practice suggests that a discussion of interventions, including medications for possible deterioration and determination of which team members would be necessary to accompany and assist the nurse is vital to ensure patient safety.

## SEIZURE

Seizures may also be considered a cause for neurologic change; however, there is little evidence that MMCA stroke increases seizure risk more than other neurologic injuries. Bianchin and colleagues[27–29] did report a higher risk of seizure in a small sample of MMCA stroke patients post-DHC. EEG and seizure prophylaxis decisions would be determined appropriate by the ICU team. If seizure is suspected, long-term EEG monitoring for 24 hours or longer may be applied as a seizure rule-out strategy.

## INTRACRANIAL PRESSURE MONITORING

Clinical deterioration from an MMCA stroke is caused by displacement and shifting of the hypothalamus and brainstem and therefore may not display an elevation of global ICP. Poca and colleagues[30] found patients with MMCA stroke showed clinical deterioration without change to ICP, which has influenced overall management and hemicraniectomy decisions. The early use of ICP monitoring in hemispheric strokes is not recommended.[18] There is, however, a pudicity of evidence about the use of ICP monitoring later in the course of the patient's clinical care, and decisions about its use are often left to the clinical team. If ICP monitoring is being used the nurse should be vigilant in maintaining positioning that promotes venous outflow and minimizes herniation risk. The optimal HOB position has not been determined but best practice dictates HOB elevation of at least 30° assists in maintaining venous outflow. Keeping the patient's head in a neutral position enhances jugular outflow.[18,20] Using reverse

Trendelenburg to raise the HOB aides in avoiding hip flexion greater than 60°, which may also decrease venous outflow.[23]

## HEMODYNAMICS

Cerebral hemorrhage may be a risk if MMCA patients are hypertensive, received thrombolytics, or are post-EVT; however, there are no data to support one specific BP goal. Standard BP goals used to manage patients post-procedure are recommended. Hypertension (systolic BP >220 mm Hg or diastolic BP >105 mm Hg) is associated with increased risk of hemorrhagic conversion in patients post-stroke.[18,31] Antihypertensive medications commonly used in the ICU setting include labetalol, and nicardipine, which are titrated using standard ICU, American Stroke Association (ASA), and Neurocritical Care Society (NCS) guidelines. Nipride and hydralazine are often avoided because of vasodilatory properties and concerns related to ICP.[19]

Euvolemia is maintained to aid in BP management and isotonic solutions; such as, 0.9% normal saline are recommended for hypotension.[18,32] Common ICU vasoconstrictive agents include, norepinephrine (Levophed) or phenylephrine (Neosynephrine) titrated to a BP goal. Patients with MMCA stroke are monitored for arrhythmias per acute ASA and NCS stroke guidelines. Continuous electrocardiogram monitoring, evaluation of rate and rhythm, and electrolyte (potassium, magnesium, phosphorous, calcium) replacement is managed per ICU clinical care standards.[19]

## GLUCOSE CONTROL

Hyperglycemia is associated with worsening edema and increased risk of hemorrhagic conversion.[33,34] Blood glucose is managed according to current acute stroke ASA and NCS guidelines with target goals of 140 to 180 mg/dL.[18,19] Trials of glyburide (a sulfonylurea), which inhibits sulfonylurea receptor 1, a receptor that plays a role in the development of edema and reduces secondary injury, has shown promise in interfering with edema formation in MMCA stroke.[33] More data are needed before use in the management of MMCA stroke.

## TEMPERATURE MANAGEMENT

Fever occurs in 40% to 60% of stroke patients and is associated with increased infarct size and poor outcomes. Fever contributes to an increase of the cerebral metabolic rate modifying the production of free radicals and glutamate, and increases the risk of cerebral edema in MMCA patients.[18,35,36] Aggressive targeted temperature management is recommended to control fever and minimize secondary injury using normothermia targets of 36.5°C (97.7°F) to 37.5°C (99.5°F).[37] The use of a normothermia guideline is key in reducing patient risk related to the manipulation of body temperature that may include hypotension, bradycardia, and shivering leading to increased cerebral metabolism, increased cerebral edema, and ICP.[36] The guideline should describe the desired temperature goal, identification of a continuous temperature measurement device with continuous feedback loop that maintains a target temperature and ensures the safe delivery of therapy. The nurse should use a beside shiver scale to assess the patient at least every 30 minutes to 1 hour for presence or absence of shivering (**Table 1**). Common pharmacologic interventions used to decrease shivering include acetaminophen, buspirone, magnesium sulfate, meperidine, dexmedetomidine, propofol, or cistaticurium.[36] Decision to discontinue targeted temperature management is based on risk/benefit. Hypothermia has been considered

| Table 1 | |
|---|---|
| **Bedside shivering assessment scale** | |
| Score | Definition |
| 0 | None: no shivering noted on palpation of the masseter, neck, or chest wall |
| 1 | Mild: shivering localized to the neck and/or thorax only |
| 2 | Moderate: shivering involves gross movement of the upper extremities (in addition to neck and thorax) |
| 3 | Severe: shivering involves gross movements of the trunk and upper and lower extremities |

*From* Badjatia N, Strongilis E, Gordon E, et al. Metabolic impact of shivering during therapeutic temperature modulation: the Bedside Shivering Assessment Scale. Stroke 2008;39(12):3243; with permission.

for use in MMCA management and has been used on a case-by-case basis; however, there are little data to support its use at this time and more research is needed before a recommendation may be made.[9]

## HYPEROSMOLAR THERAPY

There are insufficient data to recommend hyperosmolar therapy prophylactically in MMCA stroke and use may promote reversal of the osmotic gradients leading to rebound cerebral edema and ICP.[9,18] There is also a lack of evidence about its use in MMCA stroke once clinical deterioration occurs. The clinical team may choose to use mannitol or hypertonic saline as a rescue strategy or as a bridge to hemicraniectomy, despite the data and given the lack of other effective therapies. Mannitol dosing is weight based at 1 g/kg and delivered rapidly within 20 to 30 minutes for optimum benefit. Calculation of the osmolarity gap assists in determining renal clearance for continued dosing strategies.[32] If 23.4% hypertonic saline is preferred, it is delivered via central line access in a bolus dose over 10 to 30 minutes. In an acute, emergent situation, a large-bore peripheral line is appropriate and if continued administration is desired a central line is required. The patient should be monitored for the development of pulmonary edema, a common side effect of continued 23.4% dosing.[32] Other ICP management interventions, such as corticosteroids and barbiturates, have not improved outcome and are not recommended.[19]

## DECOMPRESSIVE HEMICRANIECTOMY

The risk of malignant edema in MMCA patients requires the clinical team to discuss the need for decompressive craniectomy, also referred to as hemicraniectomy. DHC has been supported as the one intervention that increases survival and has the possibility to improve outcome with those patients younger than 60 years of age.[38] Timing of the procedure is critical, however, and the risks associated with surgery discourage prophylactic surgical intervention.[18] Early DHC, within 24 to 48 hours after the onset of symptoms, has demonstrated lower mortality and better outcomes, whereas surgery performed greater than 72 hours did not improve the odds of a good outcome. More data are needed before optimal surgical timing can be determined.[39] The STATE criteria acronym (*S*core, *T*ime, *A*ge, *T*erritory, *E*xpectations), is an example of a clinical decision tool representing the pooled analysis of three randomized controlled trials supporting DHC and used to guide physicians in DHC decision-making (**Table 2**).[11]

| Table 2 | |
|---|---|
| **STATE acronym for inclusion criteria from pooled analysis of major randomized trials of craniectomy in middle cerebral artery** | |
| **Factor** | **Criteria** |
| Score | NIHSS item 1a $\geq$1 and NIHSS score >15 |
| Time | Within 45 h of after onset of symptoms (ie, 48 h to treatment) |
| Age | 18–60 y |
| Territory | Infarct lesion volume >145 cm$^3$ on diffusion-weighted MRI or signs on CT of an infarct at least 50% of MCA territory, with or without additional infarction in the territory of anterior or posterior cerebral artery on same side (volume is estimated by simple method) |
| Expectations | Written informed consent from patient or legal representative; in our practice, we emphasize that informed consent should include understanding that decompressive craniectomy improves survival but patients can still have significant disability |

*From* Agarwalla PK, Stapleton CJ, Ogilvy CS. Craniectomy in acute ischemic stroke. Neurosurgery. 2014;74 Suppl 1;S155; with permission.

If DHC is performed, postoperative ICU care includes continued neurologic assessment and hemodynamic monitoring with a BP goal of less than 140 mm Hg to reduce the risk of hemorrhagic transformation in the first 24 to 48 hours post-procedure; then the BP goal is at the team's discretion based on clinical response. Additional postoperative risks include infection, seizure, and cerebral spinal fluid leak.[6] The craniectomy flap is assessed each shift. A taut or tight flap implies edema and pressure, whereas a "boggy" or soft flap implies less edema and less pressure being exerted. Patients are on "flap precautions" and pressure on the flap is avoided. Patients may be turned, and neck positioned with a towel to encourage pressure relief and to maintain alignment[6] and signage cautioning other team members, including family, to position restrictions is helpful in maintaining patient safety. The patient is at risk for fall because of their overall neurologic condition and a helmet is used when a patient is mobilized out of bed.[13] Complications that may occur later in the postoperative period include "sunken flap syndrome," and subgaleal fluid collection. Sunken flap occurs as edema subsides and the skin sinks into the craniectomy site. Trendelenburg positioning (supine position tilted down at 15°–30°) and/or surgical replacement of the flap are two treatment interventions. Postoperatively, fluid or blood may build in the subgaleal space found between the scalp and the skull and causing pressure in the surgical site. If a subgaleal collection is present, a small drain may be placed to provide decompression.[11] Decision to perform a cranioplasty to return the missing bone flap is made by the neurosurgical team and depends on the GOC. There is no evidence to guide the best time for cranioplasty, although it usually occurs at 8 to 10 weeks if the patient is free of infection.

One of the most important considerations when considering DHC is obtaining consent from the patient or the surrogate decision maker. DHC is considered a life-saving procedure, most often requiring rapid decision-making; however, surgical decompression may still result in high morbidity, especially for those older than 60 years of age.[40] There is no guarantee that patients post-DHC will have good functional recovery.[41] The nurse is in a pivotal role as a patient advocate and should take the lead in arranging a GOC meeting with the family. Discussion should focus on the high probability that the patient will survive, although there is uncertainty regarding residual functional abilities and the possibility of total dependence on others for all their care. What would the patient say if he or she knew about dependency and disability? In quality of life studies to date, most DHC patients, with or without impairments, and their caregivers, were asked if they would choose DHC again. Despite outcomes most responded "yes." The variables identified as influencing their decision-making included severity of disability, premorbid lifestyle, patient personality, and relationship to his or her relatives.[42]

### Case example

A 46-year-old man with left MMCA stroke was admitted to the neurologic ICU with a reported NIHSS of 19 (0–42), indicating significant disability. Head CT demonstrated edema and an ASPECTS score estimated at seven. He was arousable, opened eyes to voice or slight touch, pupils equal at 4 mm and brisk, localizing with right side to superficial nail bed pain. The patient's wife met with the neurologic ICU team, and the nurse reinforced teaching demonstrating the examination and discussing possible deterioration. At hour 16, the patient demonstrated a decreased LOC on examination; pupils were anisocoric, left 5 mm and sluggish and right 4 mm and brisk. The right arm was now flexing to deep painful stimuli. Expedited CT demonstrated increased edema greater than 50% of the left hemispheric territory as compared with the prior CT (**Fig. 5**). The patient received 23.4% hypertonic saline. His wife, acting as surrogate decision maker, consented to surgery. "He would want us to do everything even if he couldn't be the same," and patient was taken to the operating room for a DHC (**Fig. 6**). He returned to the unit intubated, posthemicraniectomy, flap slightly taut, hemodynamically stable, with an improved examination of pupils now equal and reactive, again purposefully withdrawing his right arm to nail bed pain.

### PATIENT AND FAMILY SUPPORT

The patient with an MMCA stroke is a high-risk admission, the course of care is complex, and the outcome uncertain. The role of the nurse in guiding the family throughout the hospitalization cannot be underestimated. The patient and/or the family are in crisis on arrival and will be making life-saving or life-changing decisions. Developing relationships that aid in guiding and advocating for the patient begin on admission. Sharing knowledge, "getting to know" the patient and family

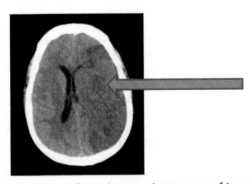

**Fig. 5.** Increased edema LMCA territory. Arrow points to area of increased edema causing brain shift.

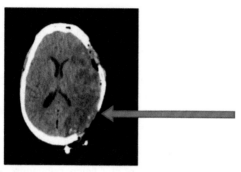

**Fig. 6.** CT scan post hemicraniectomy. Arrow points to Case study: Post craniectomy with, edema and shift improved.

including values and beliefs, promoting self-care, arranging family meetings, and communicating the daily plan of care or changes in condition helps to foster trust in caregivers. Encouraging family presence at the bedside to demystify care and demonstrate nursing vigilance and providing gentle boundaries are some techniques that aid in crisis management.[38,43] Any nurse advocating for the patient should have knowledge of pathophysiology, management strategies, and possible outcomes that aid in educating the patient and family. Patients with MMCA stroke have high morbidity and mortality despite aggressive interventions. GOC and end-of-life decisions are part of the process. A consultation to the organ procurement organization should be made if the patient's condition worsens and a palliative approach is desired by the surrogate decision maker.[44] It is important for the nurse to have knowledge of quality of life and neuroprognostication. In studies about quality of life, caregivers and patients revealed that despite poor outcomes their quality of life was acceptable. Only one-third of these patients' physicians thought the outcome was desirable suggesting that other factors identified as social, financial, or resiliency itself played a role in patient or family satisfaction. Nursing and team resiliency are often tested in these high-risk situations and organizing ethics rounds, collaborative case reviews, and mindfulness exercises for the team are some best practice strategies that contribute to ensuring an environment of caring and support for the ICU staff.

## SUMMARY

MMCA stroke management continues to be a challenge despite studies that have contributed to evaluation and treatment. Establishment of EVT that benefits reperfusion and data supporting the use of DHC has aided in improving outcomes. Continued areas of research include predicting patients at risk for herniation, management strategies that can reduce or prevent edema formation, technology to assist in monitoring, and patient outcome studies.

The patient and family need information and support that help them during the acute care period and to prepare for the road ahead. The nurse plays a vital role in providing care, knowledge, and support that is needed for critical decision making by the patient, family, and team.

## DISCLOSURE

The author has nothing to disclose.

## REFERENCES

1. Huttner HB, Schwab S. Malignant middle cerebral artery infarction: clinical characteristics, treatment strategies, and future perspectives. Lancet Neurol 2009; 8(10):949–58.
2. Qureshi A. Timing of neurologic deterioration in massive middle cerebral artery infarction: a multicenter review. Crit Care Med 2003;3(1):272–7.
3. Rastogi V, Lamb D, Williamson JB. Hemispheric differences in malignant middle cerebral artery stroke. J Neurosciences 2015;353:20–7.
4. Meyer S, Strattmatter M, Fischer C. Lateralization in autonomic dysfunction in ischemic stroke involving the insular cortex. Neuroreport 2004;15(2):357–61.
5. Lauritzen M, Dreier J, Fabricius M, et al. Clinical relevance of cortical spreading depression in neurological disorders: migraine, malignant stroke, subarachnoid and intracranial hemorrhage, and traumatic brain injury. J Cereb Blood Flow Metab 2011;31:17–35.
6. Heiss W. Malignant MCA infarction: pathophysiology and imaging for early diagnosis and management decisions. Cerebrovasc Dis 2016;41:1–7.
7. MacCallum C, Churilov L, Mitchell P, et al. Low Alberta stroke program early CT score (Aspects) associated with malignant middle cerebral artery infarction. Cerebrovasc Dis 2014;38:39–45.
8. Broocks G, Hanning U, Flottmann F, et al. Clinical benefit of thrombectomy in stroke patients with low aspects is mediated by oedema reduction. Brain 2009; 142(5):1399–407.
9. Maciel C, Sheth K. Malignant MCA stroke: an update on surgical decompression and future directions. Curr Atheroscler Rep 2015;17:40.
10. Wu S, Yuan R, Wang Y. Early prediction of malignant brain edema after ischemic stroke. A systematic review and meta-analysis. Stroke 2018;49:2918–27.
11. Agarwalla P, Stapleton C, Ogilvy C. Craniectomy in acute stroke. Neurosurgery 2014;74:S151–62.
12. Fuhrer H, Schonenberger S, Niesen W, et al. Endovascular stroke treatment's impact on malignant type of edema (ESTIMATE). J Neurol 2019;266:223–31.
13. Donovan A, Aldrich J, Matthew M, et al. Interprofessional care and teamwork in the ICU. Crit Care Med 2018;46(6):980–90.
14. Epstein N. Multidisciplinary in-house hospital team improves patient outcome: a review. Spine 2014;5(7):S295–303.
15. Bershad E, Feen E, Hernandez O, et al. Impact of specialized neurointensive care team on outcomes of critically ill acute ischemic stroke patients. Neurocrit Care 2008;9(3):287–92.
16. Shah S, Yu K, Ricon F, et al. Neurocritical critical care services influence following large hemispheric infarction and their impact on resource utilization. J Crit Care Med (Targu Mures) 2018;4(1):5–11.
17. Walcott B, Kamel H, Castrol B, et al. Tracheostomy following sever ischemic stroke: a population-based study. J Cerebrovasc Dis 2014;23(50):1024–9.
18. Wijdicks EFM, Sheth KN, Carter BS, et al, on behalf of the American Heart Association Stroke Council. Recommendations for the management of cerebral and cerebellar infarction with swelling: a statement for healthcare professionals from the American Heart Association/American Stroke Association. Stroke 2014;45: 1222–38.
19. Brogan M, Manno E. Treatment of malignant brain edema and increased intracranial pressure after stroke. Curr Treat Options Neurol 2015;17:327.

20. Hinkle J, Siewert L, Morrison K, et al. Chapter 12 ischemic stroke. In: Bader M, Littlejohns L, Olsen D, editors. Core curriculum of neuroscience nurses. 6th edition. Chicago: American Association of Neuroscience Nurses; 2016. p. 229–46.
21. Blacker D, Wijdicks E. Delayed complete bilateral ptosis associated with massive infarction of the right hemisphere. Mayo Clin Proc 2003;78:836–9.
22. Hinkle J, Morrison K, Stewert L. Chapter 12 ischemic stroke. In: Bader M, Littlejohns L, Olson D, editors. AANN core curriculum for neuroscience nursing. Chicago: American Association of Neuroscience Nurses; 2016. p. 229–46.
23. Madden L, Lewis L, Puccio A. Chapter 9 intracranial pressure management. In: Bader M, Littlejohns L, Olson D, editors. AANN core curriculum for neuroscience nursing. Chicago: American Association of Neuroscience Nurses; 2016. p. 185–203.
24. Oddo M, Crippa I, Mehta S. Optimizing sedation in patients with acute brain injury. Crit Care 2016;20:128.
25. Harvey M, Davidson J, Stollings J, et al. Post intensive care syndrome: right care, right now. Crit Care Med 2016;44(2):381–5.
26. Berlin T, Cecil S, Olin K, et al. Chapter 7 technology. In: Bader M, Littlejohns L, Olson D, editors. AANN core curriculum for neuroscience nursing. Chicago: American Association of Neuroscience Nurses; 2016. p. 163–4.
27. Bianchin M, Brondani R, deAlmeida A, et al. Seizures and epilepsy after decompressive hemicraniectomy for malignant middle cerebral artery stroke. J Neurol Sci 2017;381:336.
28. Zweckberger L, Juettler E, Bosel J, et al. Surgical aspects of decompression craniectomy in malignant stroke: review. Cerebrovasc Dis 2014;38:313–23.
29. Livesay S, Moser H. Evidence based nursing review of craniectomy. Stroke 2014; 45:217–9.
30. Poca MA, Benejam B, Sahuquillo J, et al. Monitoring intracranial pressure in patients with malignant middle cerebral artery infarction: is it useful? J Neurosurg 2010;112(3):648–57.
31. de Courten-Myers GM, Kleinholz M, Holm P, et al. Hemorrhagic infarct conversion in experimental stroke. Ann Emerg Med 1992;21:120–6.
32. Kimberly T, Sheth K. Approach to severe hemispheric stroke. Neurology 2011;76: S50–6.
33. Sheth KN, Elm JJ, Molyneaux BJ, et al. Safety and efficacy of intravenous glyburide on brain swelling after large hemispheric infarction (GAMES-RP): a randomized, double-blind18., placebo-controlled phase 2 trial. Lancet Neurol 2016;15: 1160–9.
34. van Middelaar T, Nederkoorn P, van der Worp H, et al. Quality of life after surgical decompression for space-occupying middle cerebral artery infarction: systematic review. Int J Stroke 2015;10(2):170–6.
35. Greer D, Funk S, Reaven N. Impact of fever on outcome in patients with stroke and neurologic injury a comprehensive meta-analysis. Stroke 2008;39:3029–35.
36. Guanci M, Matthiesen C. Chapter 8 temperature management. In: Bader M, Littlejohns L, Olson D, editors. AANN Core curriculum for neuroscience nursing. Chicago: American Association of Neuroscience Nurses; 2016. p. 169–82.
37. Andrews P, Verma V, Healey M, et al. Targeted temperature management in patients with intracerebral hemorrhage, subarachnoid hemorrhage, and acute ischemic stroke: a consensus recommendation. Br J Anaesth 2018;121(4): 768–75.
38. Calvin A, Kite-Powell D, Hickey J. The neuroscience ICU nurse's perceptions about end-of-life care. J Neurosci Nurs 2007;39(3):143–50.

39. Vahedi K, Hofmeijer J, Juettler E, et al. Early decompressive surgery in malignant infarction of the middle cerebral artery: a pooled analysis of three randomized controlled trials. Lancet Neurol 2007;6:215–22.
40. Das S, Mitchell P, Ross N. Decompressive hemicraniectomy in the treatment of malignant middle cerebral artery infarction: a meta-analysis. World Neurosurg 2019;123:8–16.
41. Pandhi A, Tsivgoulis G, Goyal N, et al. Hemicraniectomy for malignant middle cerebral artery syndrome: a review of functional outcomes in two high-column stroke centers. J Stroke Cerebrovasc Dis 2018;27(9):2405–10.
42. Weil A, Rahme R, Moumdjian R, et al. Quality of life following hemicraniectomy for malignant MCA territory infarction. Can J Neurol Sci 2011;38:434–8.
43. Hwang D, Yadoga D, Perry M, et al. Consistency of communication among intensive care unit staff as perceived by family members of patients surviving to discharge. J Crit Care 2014;29(1):134–8.
44. Cai X, Robinson J, Muehlschlegel S, et al. Patient preference and surrogate decision making in neurointensive care units. Neurocrit Care 2015;1:131–41.

# Priority Nursing Interventions Caring for the Stroke Patient

Mary P. Amatangelo, DNP, RN, ACNP-BC, CCRN, CNRN, SCRN, FAHA[a],*,
Sarah Beth Thomas, MSN, RN, CCRN, SCRN, CNRN[b]

## KEYWORDS

- Complex ischemic stroke patients • Intensive care unit (ICU) nursing care
- Poststroke complications

## KEY POINTS

- It is estimated that 20% of all patients with ischemic stroke (IS) will require management in an intensive care unit (ICU), particularly those treated with intravenous (IV) alteplase or endovascular therapy.
- Nursing diligence and ICU monitoring improve patient outcomes and reduce disability.
- A collaborative interdisciplinary team approach is instrumental in the ICU care of acute stroke patients.

## INTRODUCTION

It is estimated that approximately 30% of all ischemic stroke (IS) patients will deteriorate in the first 24 hours regardless of pharmacologic and/or mechanical intervention (eg, mechanical thrombectomy, endovascular thrombectomy, intraarterial mechanical thrombectomy).[1,2] Nurses play a vital role as members of the interdisciplinary care team in the management of the acute stroke patient along the continuum. Key nursing functions while caring for the acute stroke patient include, coordinating interdisciplinary team activities, preventing complications, along with educating and supporting the patient and family.

During the acute phase of stroke care, the nurse will monitor airway, breathing, and circulation (ABCs). Early assessment for neurologic compromise should be ongoing for acute stroke patients are at considerable risk for hemorrhagic transformation (HT), cerebral edema (brain swelling), and secondary strokes.[3] Essential nursing interventions include, preventing hypoxemia, blood pressure (BP) management, arrhythmia detection, particularly for atrial fibrillation (AFib), treating hyper and hypoglycemia, pulmonary and urinary tract infections (UTI) and monitoring for malnutrition and skin breakdown.[3]

---

[a] Neurology, Stroke, Neurocritical Care, Brigham and Women's Hospital, 15 Francis Street, BB 335, Boston, MA 02115, USA; [b] Neuroscience/Critical Care, Brigham Health/Brigham and Women's Hospital, 75 Francis Street, Tower 10-65, Boston, MA 02115, USA
* Corresponding author.
*E-mail address:* MAMATANGELO@BWH.HARVARD.EDU

Crit Care Nurs Clin N Am 32 (2020) 67–84
https://doi.org/10.1016/j.cnc.2019.11.005
0899-5885/20/© 2019 Elsevier Inc. All rights reserved.

Given the complexity of an acute stroke patient, and the potential complications, an interdisciplinary care team composed of a critical care intensivist, neurologist, neurosurgeon, nurse, physical, occupational, speech, and respiratory therapist, and dietician is optimal to clinically manage patients with stroke successfully. Patients receiving specialized stroke care have statistically better outcomes, 17% to 28% reduction in death, 7% increase in the ability to live at home, and 5% reduction in length of stay.[2,4-6]

## AFTER ALTEPLASE AND ENDOVASCULAR THROMBECTOMY

Approximately, 10% of acute ischemic strokes (AIS) will deteriorate due to progression of cerebral ischemia, 10% for cerebral edema, and more than 3% related to a secondary insult or HT.[2,7] The progression of AIS is influenced by several factors including, the rate of stroke onset, duration of ischemia, the integrity of collateral circulation, adequate systemic circulation, hematologic causes, elevated body temperature, and the presence of hypoglycemia/hyperglycemia.[8]

In the first few hours of an AIS (<24 hours), there are 3 stages of cerebral tissue injury: the infarcted core, the ischemic penumbra, and the oligemic region (areas of reduced vascular flow).[8,9] The penumbra is the target of acute intervention. Timely restoration of cerebral blood flow (CBF) using reperfusion therapy, IV alteplase, and/or endovascular thrombectomy are the most effective time-sensitive interventions for salvaging ischemic brain tissue.[10] The infarcted core will progressively recruit the ischemic penumbra, leading to the concept of "time is brain."[9] or the "window of opportunity."[8] The penumbra is a viable area and can be partially or completely reversed if reperfusion occurs; though, the benefit of reperfusion decreases overtime.[8,9]

The American Heart Association/American Stroke Association (AHA/ASA) 2019 Guidelines for the Early Management of Patients with Acute Ischemic Stroke, advocate that patients who receive IV alteplase or endovascular thrombectomy be admitted to an ICU for post procedure management of neurologic deficits, bleeding complications, and control of hemodynamic variability.[2,11-13]

## BLEEDING ASSESSMENT

IV alteplase is first-line therapy for AIS, and is required to be administered within 4.5 hours of symptom onset. IV thrombolysis increases the risk of HT into the infarcted

---

**Box 1**
**Recommended bleeding precautions (24 hours from alteplase start time)[123,124]**

- Arterial and venous puncture sites should be minimized and checked frequently
- Avoid or defer bladder catheterizations, or nasogastric tube placement unless medically necessary
- No pharmacological deep vein thrombosis (DVT) prophylaxis
- Bed rest for 8 hours after alteplase administration and then advance activity as tolerated under direct nursing supervision
- Monitor for signs of petechial hemorrhages under bilateral knee–high sequential compression devices and noninvasive blood pressure (NBP) cuffs in use
- Rotation of NBP cuff recommended a minimum of every 2 hours

cerebral tissue. In the first 12 to 24 hours after IV alteplase, monitoring for bleeding is a critical function of the ICU nurse (**Box 1**).

During an AIS, core necrotic tissue exists and varies in composition. A larger area of infarction results in increased intracellular edema, erratic amounts of congestion owing to blood vessel dilation, and extravasation of blood and other cells. This creates softened fragile tissue, further compromising adequate blood supply before stabilizing between 24 to 72 hours.[8–10,14] The larger the infarcted territory, the greater the risk of secondary injury.

Age, stroke severity, hypertension, atrial fibrillation (AFib), anticoagulation, such as warfarin (regardless of prothrombin time), and hyperglycemia are contributing factors to HT in patients with AIS treated with IV alteplase.[15] Studies report 30% to 40% of patients with AIS will have intracranial HT.[3,7,16] Any variance in the bedside neurologic exam, using the National Institutes of Health Stroke Scale (NIHSS),[1,8,16] warrants repeat non contrast head CT.

The use of IV alteplase also increases the risk of bleeding complications outside the brain. The nurse should monitor for oozing and bleeding orally (gums), hemoptysis, arterial and venipuncture sites, hematuria, and scattered ecchymosis. Bleeding precautions are implemented when considering alteplase (**Box 2**).[11,17]

In addition to, or independent of IV alteplase, mechanical thrombectomy, or clot retrieval, is indicated for patients with AIS presenting with a large vessel occlusion (LVO). Patients eligible for mechanical thrombectomy may or may not have already received IV alteplase for the same ischemic stroke event and should be intervened upon with 24 hours of last known well (LKW).[10,11]

Vascular access and sheath options are available to the interventionalist when performing percutaneous transcatheter procedures. Commonly used access sites include radial or femoral arteries.[17] Post procedure, patients should arrive to the ICU with a knee immobilizer applied to the groin puncture site leg.[4,18] Additional nursing assessment post procedure is required for monitoring the sheath site for bleeding and hematoma formation and for assessing pulses of the bilateral lower extremities, focusing on the dorsalis pedis (DP) and posterior tibial (PT) pulses along with capillary refill.[11]

The post procedure limb should not have a sequential compression device applied until bed rest is completed. Bed rest and keeping the head of the bed (HOB) flat, post procedure, are routinely implemented for 4 to 6 hours with direct nursing supervision for advancement in activity and HOB elevation. Nursing assessment at this time is focused on the potential formation of a groin site hematoma, and groin site bleeding.

It is an emergency if at any point post procedure the puncture site suddenly begins to bleed, or the distal pulses of the post procedure limb diminish. The physician should be notified immediately, while the nurse applies pressure to the bleeding site. If distal

---

**Box 2**
**Selected signs and symptoms of hemorrhagic transformation**[7,9,12]

- Elevation of blood pressure
- Weakness or sudden deterioration of motor examination in any extremity, particularly the already effected limb
- Onset of new headache
- Nausea and/or vomiting
- Altered level of consciousness

pulses are absent, an emergent ultrasound (US) should be performed. The patient and family should be prepared for a potential interventional procedure.[19,20]

## BLOOD PRESSURE (BP) MANAGEMENT

Initially post AIS, there is a transient hypertensive effect in 60% of all AIS within the first 48 hours.[8–11] BP variability in the first 24 hours is independently associated with increasing neurologic deterioration and an increase in intracranial pressure (ICP) that can lead to secondary brain injury. Secondary brain injury occurs as an indirect result of the primary injury, in this instance, AIS. The development is gradual in nature and involves an array of cellular processes, often preventable and modifiable. It can be associated with the primary acute stroke or independent of it. Common examples include cerebral edema (swelling), cerebral hypoxia (insufficient oxygen to the brain), altered cerebral blood flow (CBF), hematoma expansion, ischemia, or HT.[21–23]

BP management according to the recommended AHA/ASA 2019 Guidelines for patients with AIS who are, both eligible, and not, candidates for IV alteplase as well as hemorrhagic strokes (**Box 3**).[1,13,18,24] If systemic BP is elevated, there is a 50% increased risk of recurrent IS or HT.[25,26] Specific to this is, if BP is too low, creating hypoperfusion, there is an increased risk of compromising collateral blood flow and expanding the existing infarction.[25,26] Patients with AIS with a systolic blood pressure (SBP) less than 140 mm Hg throughout their hospitalization, and at discharge, are at significant risk of mortality, and increased morbidity.[27,28] It is important to note, there is limited research clarifying this.[27–31]

Continued evaluation of factors contributing to elevated BP should be assessed by the ICU nurse. Factors include physiologic responses to hypoxia, preexisting hypertension, increased ICP, HT, pain, nausea, and noise levels.[1,4,25,32,33] The physician may place a radial arterial line to assist in BP monitoring. An arterial line is valuable in the ICU stroke patient for continuous BP monitoring and frequent lab draws. These are patients with sub-occluded vessels, cerebral stenosis, vasospasm, hydrocephalus and uncontrolled hypertension requiring pharmacologic agents to decrease or increase BP (**Box 4**).[34–36]

Hypotension, or hypoperfusion, is less common in the AIS patient. Hypovolemia should be considered while assessing hypotension in patients with known subocclusive vessels, myocardial ischemia (MI), or cardiac arrhythmias which decrease cardiac output (CO), and systemic perfusion required to maintain vital organ function.[13,24] There are no best practice recommendations regarding pharmacologic agents to manage low BP; however, AHA/ASA 2019 Guidelines along with the European Stroke Organization (ESO) Guidelines endorse administering normal saline (NS 0.9%) for fluid replacement.[13,24,37] Currently, there is no data or research to guide volume and duration of parenteral fluid administration as well as to compare different isotonic fluids.[13] If there is a high probability of cerebral swelling or fluid overload secondary to brain or cardiovascular injury, colloids (albumin) might be considered an alternative to crystalloids (NS 0.9%, D5 NS).[24,37]

There may be a role for further decrease in BP post endovascular procedure, with a goal to avoid potential reperfusion injury to the ischemic cerebral tissue.[16] Reperfusion injury describes a complex pathophysiologic process that may hyperperfuse already

---

**Box 3**
**Blood pressure caution**

Caution: If blood pressure exceeds 220/120 mm Hg, reduction of only 15% recommended within the first 24 hours to avoid further compromise of cerebral blood flow[32,33]

at risk ischemic tissue even after successful recanalization of an occluded vessel.[14,16] AHA/ASA 2019 Guidelines recommend maintaining BP ≤180/105 mm Hg during the first 24 hours post procedure.[13,14,24,38,39]

## CARDIAC MONITORING

Continuous cardiac monitoring during the first 24 to 72 hours after stroke is recommended based on current AHA/ASA 2019 Guidelines, however, there is currently no consensus on the optimal method or duration for monitoring after the initial 24 hours from admission.[13,24,40] Cardiac arrhythmias and abnormal electrocardiograms (EKGs) are identified in 50% to 70% of all acute stroke patients.[41] Cardiac abnormalities vary from abnormal T waves, prolonged QT intervals (often associated with drug therapy), ST segment inversions, atrial and ventricular arrhythmias, premature ventricular contractions (PVCs), tachycardia, heart blocks, and most notably, paroxysmal atrial fibrillation (PAF) (**Box 5**).[40–43] In a global survey, 28% of AIS patients had AFib.[40]

Underlying cardiac mechanisms in the setting of AIS are often not known, however, there is a direct disruption in the autonomic nervous system that unconsciously regulates body functions, such as heart rate, respiratory rate, and pupillary response.[44] It is prudent to monitor for EKG abnormalities and trend QT intervals for electrolyte imbalance, autonomic fluctuations, and medications which increase the risk of developing sudden cardiac death and secondary stroke. Cardiac arrhythmias are common in right cerebral hemispheric strokes specifically relating to the right insular cortex.[41,45]

More than 40% of AIS patients experience myocardial infarction (MI), without preexisting cardiac disease. Two-thirds of those MIs are silent. Elevated troponin levels are noted in 10% of all AIS.[44] Early positive troponins are thought independently associated with a cardiac embolic source.[15] Daily patient weight, EKGs, serum cardiac enzymes, troponin, electrolytes, including potassium, magnesium, calcium, and phosphorous, are also important to trend in the prevention of secondary cardiac ischemia and fatal arrhythmias.[4,24,40–42,45]

## TEMPERATURE

The relationship between brain function and temperature is vital. Cerebral metabolism (CM), cerebral blood flow (CBF), and permeability of the blood-brain barrier (BBB) change proportionally with brain temperature. For every degree Celsius of body temperature increase, there is a 6% to 8% increase in CM. Increasing temperature damages the endothelial cells of the brain and spinal cord, allowing diffusion through the BBB, which contributes to cerebral edema and increased intracranial pressure (ICP).[46,47]

There is a 60% incidence that the stroke patient will develop a fever.[48,49] Two-thirds of fevers are attributed to UTIs, pneumonitis, and chemical aspiration pneumonias.[48,49] Post stroke fever can also be endogenous, often referred to as "central fever" (CF).[46–49] CF are often difficult to discern from infection and are thought a response of the immune activation system, or effects of brain lesions on the thermoregulatory centers.[50]

Infectious processes typically manifest within 48 to 72 hours from onset of stroke.[46,51] Regardless of why a patient's temperature is elevated, they are more likely to die within the first 10 days after a stroke than their counterparts with normothermia.[52] Consideration of any preexisting infectious and noninfectious processes, venous thromboembolism (VTE), blood transfusion reaction, or drug administration and withdrawal would be prudent.[46,49,53] There are also negative consequences of antibiotic overuse, including adverse events, such as anaphylaxis, drug interactions, fungal infections, digestion issues, photo sensitivity, and multidrug-resistant organisms.[53]

The AHA/ASA 2019 Guidelines recommend lowering hyperthermia to normothermia 36.5°C to 37.5°C (97.7°F–99.5°F),[49] without inducing hypothermia. Hypothermia has not been proven beneficial in acute stroke.[13,24] Treating fever beginning with antipyretics is strongly advised.

## AIRWAY AND RESPIRATORY ASSESSMENT

Stroke patients with patent airways and oxygen saturation levels less than 94% should be administered supplemental oxygen.[1,16,51,54] AIS patients are frequently capable of breathing spontaneously despite persistent neurologic impairment and do not characteristically require intrusive respiratory interventions involving high-flow oxygenation, biphasic (BiPAP), or continuous positive airway pressure (CPAP).

Stroke patients who present intubated or require rapid intubation to secure a patent airway[8,54] are at risk for hypoxia as a result of inadequate cerebral tissue oxygenation and advancement of neurologic compromise related to the disruption of the autonomic nervous system. Injury, infarction, or ischemia to the posterior cerebral circulation or vertebrobasilar arteries, including the midbrain, pons, and medulla, are in jeopardy of compromising the airway for these areas regulate cardiac and respiratory function and are pivotal in maintaining consciousness.[1,8,16,54] Patients with stroke requiring intubation and mechanical ventilation have mortalities as high as 71%. Statistically, at least three-quarters of all strokes occur in people over the age of 65, which attributes to age-related respiratory mechanisms failing or were weakened at baseline.[1,55,56]

Once intubated and mechanically ventilated, it is prudent to assess the ongoing capability of the patient to oxygenate and ventilate successfully. Nursing, often in collaboration with respiratory therapy, plays a vital role in preventive care, including maintaining the HOB at 30°; assessing quality and quantity of endotracheal and oral secretions, the ability and strength of cough, and pulmonary toileting; repositioning the endotracheal tube with frequent oral care to prevent mucosal skin breakdown; turning and repositioning the patient every 2 hours with chest physiotherapy; and preventing ventilator-associated pneumonia (VAP).[1,8,24,57]

Failure to extubate the patient with AIS in a timely manner is as high as 40%, leading to increased days of mechanical ventilation, increased risk of pneumonia, increased ICU and hospital lengths of stay, and increased hospital mortality.[54] Conventional success of extubation has historically relied on level of consciousness (LOC), ability to follow commands, facial weakness, and respiratory function, including minimal ventilatory settings, presence of a cuff leak to rule out tracheal edema, strong cough, minimal endotracheal or oral secretions, and auscultation of clear lung sounds. However, liberating patients with stroke from mechanical ventilation is often challenging because of the heterogeneity of the underlying disease process.[4,19,58,59]

Extubation success in patients with stroke has been strongly correlated with younger age, location, and severity of brain injury (nonposterior circulating strokes or full hemispheric strokes) and preintubation dysphagia severity.[54,56,58,60,61] Due to the exclusivity of brain processes after stroke, consideration of a permanent airway, tracheostomy (trach), may be warranted. Reevaluating the patient's goals of care (GOC) at this stage is imperative. It is important to note that providing an opportunity to extubate versus the need and timing of a tracheostomy remains controversial.[56,62]

In addition to stroke location and severity, the presence of dysarthria is a significant contributing factor in the consideration of a tracheostomy.[58,62] Dysarthria is difficulty moving muscles in the mouth, face, or upper respiratory system that assists in controlling speech. Dysarthria in the presence of dysphagia (difficulty swallowing) increases the risk of airway compromise and aspiration.[8] Dysarthria can occur regardless of the severity of the stroke, with or without preserved LOC. The NIHSS systematically and quantitatively assesses for dysarthria.[62] Accepted advantages of a tracheostomy include decreased ventilator duration, decreased length of stay, airway safety, less pharyngeal and laryngeal lesions, higher patient comfort, and better oral hygiene.[62] It is still to be determined if the rate of pneumonia, mortality, and other complications have been sufficiently affected by early tracheostomy.[56,62]

## ASSESSMENT OF ASPIRATION

Poststroke dysphagia is categorized as either oropharyngeal or esophageal. In the case of oropharyngeal, there is a disruption or inability to pass food or liquid from the mouth to the pharynx/esophagus, which can result in aspiration.[1,62,63] In esophageal dysphagia, there is difficulty moving food or liquid through the esophagus into the stomach.[63] Clinical symptoms of dysphagia are varied and often misinterpreted or neglected by the average untrained bedside examiner (**Box 6**).[64,65]

Approximately half of all stroke patients with dysphagia will have an indication of aspiration and dysarthria. It is important to note that aspiration, like dysarthria, is a consequence of dysphagia and contributes to a 3-fold increase in mortality and length of stay, and a 6- to 7-fold increased risk of aspiration pneumonia. Dysphagia has a statistical recovery of 50% within the first 10 days to 3 weeks.[65–67]

Dysphasia screening should begin with a bedside clinical examination. A nursing swallow screen is performed initially on all patients with stroke before being given anything by mouth, including fluids, oral medication, or food.[13,24] There is no unanimity in a best practice tool to assess bedside swallow in patients with stroke; however, it should be initiated on admission, by a trained health care provider (HCP), ideally within 24 hours, with any significant neurologic changes, before intubation, and when clinically stable after extubation.[13,24,63]

---

**Box 6**
**Clinical symptoms of dysphagia[61,62]**

- Repetitive swallowing
- Abnormal volitional coughing
- Throat clearing
- Hoarseness
- Dysphonia
- Dysarthria
- Choking
- Facial weakness
- Aspiration
- Breathless upon oral intake
- Loss of liquid from the mouth
- Weight loss

---

Patients who fail a bedside swallow screen should be referred to the speech language pathologist (SLP) for a formal dysphagia evaluation.[63,64,67–73] Special consideration should be given to assess and optimize hydration status while a patient is nothing by mouth (NPO). NS or D5 NS maintenance fluid should be initiated until an SLP bedside evaluation is complete. In the hyperacute phase of stroke, dysphagia is estimated in up to 80% of patients, and at continued risk for aspiration and dysarthria. If determined unable to swallow, placement of a nasogastric tube (NGT) or a Dobhoff tube would be warranted to provide enteral nutrition and medication access. Nutrition should be consulted for tube feed recommendations.[24,74,75]

Early consideration of a percutaneous endoscopic gastrostomy (PEG) tube is also warranted if enteral feeding is likely for a period of time (>14 days). A PEG tube should be placed during a stable clinical phase (after 14–28 days), pending the long term GOC of the patient.[74] Initiate frequent monitoring of nasal mucosa as well as entry site for risk of skin breakdown and pressure ulcers. It is important to note abdominal discomfort and malabsorption, exacerbated by nausea, vomiting, bloating, or frequency of bowel elimination upon initiation of enteral nutrition (tube feeds).[4,8]

Most AIS patients will recover swallowing spontaneously, although up to 50% will experience varying levels of dysphagia after discharge, requiring modified diets, postural/position techniques, or swallowing maneuvers.[65,76]

## NUTRITION

Malnutrition is "a state resulting from a lack of intake of nutrition that leads to altered body composition and body cell mass leading to diminished physical and mental function and impaired clinical outcome from disease."[77] Historically, serum proteins (albumin, prealbumin, transferrin), C-reactive protein, total lymphocyte count, and total cholesterol were used to measure malnutrition. However, according the American Dietetic Association (ADA), serum proteins have a direct relationship with the inflammatory process and conditions which trigger this process (ie, stroke).[78] Without adequate nutrition assessment, or hydration, the patient is at continued risk for impaired immune system, increased weakness, increased weight loss, and skin breakdown.[1,4,18,77]

Daily weight, hydration status, and serum laboratory values (magnesium, potassium, calcium, and phosphate) are crucial in preventing secondary injury suggestive of refeeding syndrome, skin breakdown, muscle wasting, increasing risk for falls, cardiac arrhythmias, and infection. The ADA recommends administering a daily prophylactic multivitamin (for micronutrient coverage) as well as thiamine and folate (for prevention of Wernicke's encephalopathy) typically 3 days. Newly released literature from the AHA/ASA 2019 Guidelines suggest a correlation with vitamin D deficiency (check lab 25 [OH]D) after stroke and treatment of this if warranted.[74,78,79]

## GLUCOSE MONITORING AND CONTROL

The brain represents approximately 2% of total body weight (TBW) and uses 20% of the body's total oxygen supply and 60% of its glucose.[46] Hyperglycemia is defined as blood sugar greater than 150 mg/dL regardless if diabetic or nondiabetic.[1,44] All diabetic patients and approximately 50% to 60% of all nondiabetic patients with stroke will present with hyperglycemia in the acute phase, especially in severe strokes and those involving the insular cortex.[44,80]

Hyperglycemia is a sympathomimetic stress response and can exacerbate neurologic injury via multiple mechanisms related to increased cellular acidosis and post inflammatory responses, weakened and damaged blood vessels and nerves, contribute to plaque formation (atherosclerosis),[1] increase the risk of HT after alteplase administration, and contribute to increased mortality and hospital length of stay.[4,8,46,80]

Glycemic control within a targeted range of 140 to 180 mg/dL is a judicial approach to management in the acute phase.[4,8] If a patient has been on a home regimen of an oral or subcutaneous insulin, it is best to use either a more frequent short-acting sliding scale or a continuous insulin drip. Consider dextrose containing IV fluid (D5 NS) if patient is NPO. The goal is moderate glycemic control to reduce the risk of hypoglycemia, and avoid variability of peaks and valleys in their blood sugars.[8,11,13,24]

## SEIZURE

Not every patient with stroke will experience a seizure; that said, the ICU nurse caring for patients post stroke should be astute to the fact that both ischemic and hemorrhagic strokes account for 10% of poststroke seizures (PSS). 39% to 45% of PSS are in those older than 60 years.[81] Hemorrhagic strokes that involve the cerebral cortex (outer layer of the brain) are at greater risk of presenting with PSS.[80–82] Additional risk factors making the poststroke patient vulnerable to seizure would be the severity of the initial neurologic deficit (size of stroke, bleed, and location), younger patients less than 65 years of age, and those with a prior history of seizures.[80–82] History of alcohol (EtOH) abuse should be elicited if concern for EtOH withdrawal seizure.

PSS are classified as early or late onset.[81,83–86] Although definitions vary, early onset seizures are defined as occurring within 2 weeks of stroke and late onset seizures occurring after 2 weeks. More than half of stroke-related seizures occur in the early period. [83,87–98] Early seizures develop 73% of the time with only 26% of patients with AIS being aware of their seizures.[81]

Most seizures last less than 2.5 minutes; a prolonged seizure would be greater than 5 minutes, and status epilepticus is greater than 30 minutes. Refractory status epilepticus would be considered after the failure of 2 antiepileptic drugs (AED), and super-refractory status epilepticus would be considered after the failure of burst suppression.

There is variability in the literature establishing the value in the usefulness of providing prophylactic pharmacologic therapy in preventing or controlling seizures post stroke. Prophylactic anticonvulsants in patients with no signs or symptoms of seizure should be avoided due to low recurrence rates, and should only be considered in patients with more than 1 seizure confirmed, after stroke.[1,81,82]

Ativan IV would be the first-line agent in the hyperacute phase of seizure. Second-line, acute AEDs would be levetiracetam, lacosamide, phenytoin, valproic acid, and phenobarbital. Remember that acute AEDs may take up to 24 hours to work. An electroencephalogram (EEG) should be applied at this point. Consider an anesthetic or benzodiazepine bridge instead of adding multiple AEDs or maximizing current AED therapy. Third-line agents (burst suppression) would consider propofol, midazolam, pentobarbital, and ketamine.[99] Patients with uncontrolled seizures should be managed in a Neuro ICU for bedside EEG monitoring.

As with all critical care seizure patients, one should prioritize ABCs, observe and describe what is seen, assess LOC, eyes, pupil, gaze, head turn, tongue biting, limb shape and movement, incontinence, timing, and postictal state.

## DEEP VEIN THROMBOSIS, PROPHYLAXIS

Venous thromboembolism (VTE), including both deep vein thrombosis (DVT) and pulmonary emboli (PE) are common sequalae of stroke. DVT frequently occurs in the setting of stroke and can be a fatal complication if it leads to pulmonary emboli. The incidence of DVT vary from 10% to 75%. The onset of development of a DVT post stroke can be as early as day 2, peaking between days 2 and 7;[100,101] if untreated, proximal DVT have a 15% risk of death.[102] The prevalence of PE is 1% to 3%, which accounts for early death in the first 2 to 4 weeks after stroke onset.[103]

Risk factors for DVT in acute stroke are advanced age, female gender, high NIHSS score, hemiparesis, immobility, AFib, having received IV alteplase, and admission to an academic medical center. [104,105,106] However, immobility remains the highest contributor to the VTE risk.

The initial diagnostic test choice for peripheral venous thrombosis is ultrasound (US), due to its accuracy, low cost, portability, and safety.[107] Doppler techniques provide direct information regarding flow physiology.[108,109,110] AHA/ASA 2019 Guidelines note, immobile stroke patients without contraindications, an intermittent pneumatic compression (IPC) device in addition to routine care (aspirin and hydration) is recommended to reduce the risk of DVT.[111]

In clinical practice pharmacologic treatment can also be used for VTE prevention in patients with AIS and restricted mobility. The use of prophylactic doses of LMWH or unfractionated heparin, which should be initiated as early as possible, and continued throughout the hospital stay or until the patient has regained mobility.[112,113] This has the potential to reduce the incidence of symptomatic DVT by 70% and the incidence of fatal and nonfatal PE by 30%.[112,113]

## BLADDER BOWEL REGIMENS

Early bowel and bladder care should be initiated to prevent complications such as constipation and urinary retention or infection.[1] Bladder and bowel dysfunction after stroke affects up to 50% of all stroke survivors.[114] Urinary tract infections (UTI) affect between 10% and 19% of patients with stroke and are the most common poststroke infections owing to functional abnormalities, such as neurogenic bladder, bladder dysfunction, low cognitive function, and diminished functional level.[8,115,116] Additional risk factors for UTIs are older adults, women, higher postvoid residuals, and higher modified Rankin score.[115,116]

Assessment for bladder dysfunction should be initiated on admission and includes presence of incontinence, history of incontinence, pain or burning with urination, urgency, frequency, and previous or current UTI. If the patient presents with a Foley catheter, it would be a priority to remove it as soon as hemodynamically stable to prevent catheter associated urinary tract infection (CAUTI).[4,8,18] Hydration status, urine color, clarity, and frequency of urinary retention should be assessed if voiding independently every 8 hours or as needed. Bladder scanning, or intermittent bladder catheterization, prevoid and postvoid, can assist with determining postvoid residual volume. It is also important to subjectively assess for complaints of discomfort, pain, or burning when urinating if the patient is able to communicate.[4,18,115,116]

Constipation is a common complication post stroke. It is a major cause of morbidity and mortality in the acute and subacute phases of stroke.[117–119] The incidence of constipation in stroke patients ranges from 29% to 79%.[120] Post stroke patients with constipation are likely to experience medical complications such as pneumonia, upper GI bleeding, UTI and recurrent stroke.[121] It is important to implement a bowel regimen upon admission to the ICU. Consider a standing daily laxative (Colace) and stool softener (Senna), along with as needed (PRN) (Dulcolax) and (Miralax).

## SKIN CARE

Risk of impaired skin breakdown is significant for patients with AIS along the continuum of care. Impaired mobility, impaired circulation, altered levels of consciousness, increasing age, poor nutritional status, and dehydration along with fecal and/or urinary incontinence are contributing factors. Nursing assessment priorities include a predictive model, such as the commonly used Braden scale (predicting pressure ulcer risk) to assist in identifying the potential for skin breakdown.[4,18] By analyzing the Braden subscales and scores, 39% of hospitalized patients with cerebrovascular disease were found with limited mobility, consistent moisture, limited sensorial perception, and high risk of friction or shear forces.[4,8,114,122]

Patients need to be examined for skin breakdown and repositioned every 2 hours with special consideration to avoid excess friction or pressure.[4,18] Interdisciplinary consults, including dietary, physical, and occupational therapies, are warranted, to assist in monitoring for skin breakdown through to the rehabilitation process. Documentation of daily or more frequent Braden scale scores, mobility, and any presenting wounds is critical to prevention, especially when admitting a patient with stroke from another facility.[4,8,18,122]

## SUMMARY

Strokes represent a complex disease process. Advancements in time-sensitive treatment options require the interdisciplinary ICU care team to be in concert in the clinical management of the stroke patient and their caregivers. Nursing is a critical member of the interdisciplinary ICU team in all aspects of stroke. The expertise required of the ICU nurse in all facets of stroke management is essential in prioritizing activities of the team, preventing medical complications, providing the highest quality care, while educating, advocating and supporting the stroke patient and their family.

## DISCLOSURE

The authors have nothing to disclose.

## REFERENCES

1. Summers D, Leonard A, Wentworth D, et al. Comprehensive overview of nursing and interdisciplinary care of the acute ischemic stroke patient: a scientific statement from the American Heart Association. Stroke 2009;40(8):2911–44.
2. Becker CD, Bowers C, Chandy D, et al. Low risk monitoring in neurocritical care. Front Neurol 2018;9:938.
3. Bovim MR, Askim T, Lydersen S, et al. Complications in the first week after stroke: a 10-year comparison. BMC Neurol 2016;16(1):133.
4. Morrison K. Fast facts for stroke care nursing: an expert guide in a nutshell. 1st Edition. New York: Springer Publishing Company, LLC; 2014.
5. Morris S, Ramsay AIG, Boaden RJ, et al. Impact and sustainability of centralising acute stroke services in English metropolitan areas: retrospective analysis of hospital episode statistics and stroke national audit data. BMJ 2019;l1. https://doi.org/10.1136/bmj.l1.
6. Adeoye O, Nyström KV, Yavagal DR, et al. Recommendations for the establishment of stroke systems of care: a 2019 update: a policy statement from the American Stroke Association. Stroke 2019;50(7). https://doi.org/10.1161/STR.0000000000000173.
7. Paciaroni M, Bandini F, Agnelli G, et al. Hemorrhagic transformation in patients with acute ischemic stroke and atrial fibrillation: time to initiation of oral anticoagulant therapy and outcomes. J Am Heart Assoc 2018;7(22). https://doi.org/10.1161/JAHA.118.010133.
8. Hickey JV, Strayer A, Hickey JV, editors. The clinical practice of neurological and neurosurgical nursing. 8th edition. Philadelphia: Wolters Kluwer; 2020.
9. Gauberti M, De Lizarrondo SM, Vivien D. The "inflammatory penumbra" in ischemic stroke: from clinical data to experimental evidence. Eur Stroke J 2016;1(1):20–7.
10. Mechanical thrombectomy for acute ischemic stroke–UpToDate. Available at: https://www.uptodate.com/contents/mechanical-thrombectomy-for-acute-ischemic-stroke/print. Accessed November 4, 2019.
11. Powers WJ, Derdeyn CP, Biller J, et al. 2015 American Heart Association/American Stroke Association focused update of the 2013 guidelines for the early management of patients with acute ischemic stroke regarding endovascular treatment: a guideline for healthcare professionals from the American Heart Association/American Stroke Association. Stroke 2015;46(10):3020–35.
12. Sadaka F, Jadhav A, O'Brien J, et al. Do all acute stroke patients receiving tPA require ICU admission? J Clin Med Res 2018;10(3):174–7.
13. Powers WJ, Rabinstein AA, Ackerson T, et al. Guidelines for the early management of patients with acute ischemic stroke: 2019 update to the 2018 guidelines for the early management of acute ischemic stroke: a guideline for healthcare professionals from the American Heart Association/American Stroke Association. Stroke 2019. https://doi.org/10.1161/STR.0000000000000211.
14. Piccardi B, Arba F, Nesi M, et al. Reperfusion injury after ischemic stroke study (RISKS): single-centre (Florence, Italy), prospective observational protocol study. BMJ Open 2018;8(5):e021183.
15. Yaghi S, Chang AD, Ricci BA, et al. Early elevated troponin levels after ischemic stroke suggests a cardioembolic source. Stroke 2018;49(1):121–6.
16. Bevers MB, Kimberly WT. Critical care management of acute ischemic stroke. Curr Treat Options Cardiovasc Med 2017;19(6):41.

17. Lin L-M, Bender MT, Colby GP, et al. Use of a next-generation multi-durometer long guide sheath for triaxial access in flow diversion: experience in 95 consecutive cases. J Neurointerv Surg 2018;10(2):137–42.
18. Diepenbrock NH. Quick reference to critical care. 5th edition. Philadelphia: Wolters Kluwer; 2016.
19. Choudhury M. Postoperative management of vascular surgery patients: a brief review. Gen Surg 2017;2:1584.
20. Jadhav AP, Molyneaux BJ, Hill MD, et al. Care of the post-thrombectomy patient. Stroke 2018;49(11):2801–7.
21. Kowalski RG, Haarbauer-Krupa JK, Bell JM, et al. Acute ischemic stroke after moderate to severe traumatic brain injury: incidence and impact on outcome. Stroke 2017;48(7):1802–9.
22. Kaur P, Sharma S. Recent advances in pathophysiology of traumatic brain injury. Curr Neuropharmacol 2018;16(8):1224–38.
23. Ortega-Pérez S, Amaya-Rey MC. Secondary brain injury: a concept analysis. J Neurosci Nurs 2018;50(4):220–4.
24. Powers WJ, Rabinstein AA, Ackerson T, et al. 2018 guidelines for the early management of patients with acute ischemic stroke: a guideline for healthcare professionals from the American Heart Association/American Stroke Association. Stroke 2018;49(3). https://doi.org/10.1161/STR.0000000000000158.
25. Initial assessment and management of acute stroke–UpToDate. Available at: https://www.uptodate.com/contents/initial-assessment-and-management-of-acute-stroke?source=history_widget. Accessed July 15, 2019.
26. Tanaka E, Koga M, Kobayashi J, et al. Blood pressure variability on antihypertensive therapy in acute intracerebral hemorrhage: the stroke acute management with urgent risk-factor assessment and improvement-intracerebral hemorrhage study. Stroke 2014;45(8):2275–9.
27. Wohlfahrt P, Krajcoviechova A, Jozifova M, et al. Low blood pressure during the acute period of ischemic stroke is associated with decreased survival. J Hypertens 2015;33(2):339–45.
28. Li C, Zhang Y, Xu T, et al. Systolic blood pressure trajectories in the acute phase and clinical outcomes in 2-year follow-up among patients with ischemic stroke. Am J Hypertens 2019;32(3):317–25.
29. Hong L, Cheng X, Lin L, et al. The blood pressure paradox in acute ischemic stroke. Ann Neurol 2019;85(3):331–9.
30. Appleton JP, Sprigg N, Bath PM. Blood pressure management in acute stroke. Stroke and Vascular Neurology 2016;1:e000020.
31. Anderson CS, Huang Y, Lindley RI, et al. Intensive blood pressure reduction with intravenous thrombolysis therapy for acute ischaemic stroke (ENCHANTED): an international, randomised, open-label, blinded-endpoint, phase 3 trial. Lancet 2019;393(10174):877–88.
32. Bowry R, Navalkele DD, Gonzales NR. Blood pressure management in stroke: five new things. Neurol Clin Pract 2014;4(5):419–26.
33. Hecht JP, Richards PG. Continuous-infusion labetalol vs nicardipine for hypertension management in stroke patients. J Stroke Cerebrovasc Dis 2018;27(2):460–5.
34. Zarbiz S, Pisani M. When is a peripheral arterial catheter (A-LINE) indicated in my ICU patient? CHEST Thought Lead; 2018. Available at: https://www.chestnet.org/News/Blogs/CHEST-Thought-Leaders/2018/10/Arterial-lines. Accessed August 21, 2019.

35. Sgueglia GA, Di Giorgio A, Gaspardone A, et al. Anatomic basis and physiological rationale of distal radial artery access for percutaneous coronary and endovascular procedures. JACC Cardiovasc Interv 2018;11(20):2113–9.

36. Wallace MW, Solano JJ. Radial artery cannulation. Treasure Island, FL: StatPearls; 2019. Available at: https://www.ncbi.nlm.nih.gov/books/NBK539796/.

37. Suwanwela NC, Chutinet A, Mayotarn S, et al. A randomized controlled study of intravenous fluid in acute ischemic stroke. Clin Neurol Neurosurg 2017;161: 98–103.

38. Vitt JR, Trillanes M, Hemphill JC. Management of blood pressure during and after recanalization therapy for acute ischemic stroke. Front Neurol 2019;10:138.

39. Mistry EA, Mayer SA, Khatri P. Blood pressure management after mechanical thrombectomy for acute ischemic stroke: a survey of the StrokeNet sites. J Stroke Cerebrovasc Dis 2018;27(9):2474–8.

40. Adami A, Gentile C, Hepp T, et al. Electrocardiographic RR interval dynamic analysis to identify acute stroke patients at high risk for atrial fibrillation episodes during stroke unit admission. Transl Stroke Res 2019;10(3):273–8.

41. Ruthirago D, Julayanont P, Tantrachoti P, et al. Cardiac arrhythmias and abnormal electrocardiograms after acute stroke. Am J Med Sci 2016;351(1): 112–8.

42. Stone J, Mor-Avi V, Ardelt A, et al. Frequency of inverted electrocardiographic T waves (cerebral T waves) in patients with acute strokes and their relation to left ventricular wall motion abnormalities. Am J Cardiol 2018;121(1):120–4.

43. Scheitz JF, Nolte CH, Doehner W, et al. Stroke-heart syndrome: clinical presentation and underlying mechanisms. Lancet Neurol 2018;17(12):1109–20.

44. Zazulia AR. Critical care management of acute ischemic stroke. Contin Lifelong Learn Neurol 2009;15(3):68–82.

45. Chen Z, Venkat P, Seyfried D, et al. Brain-heart interaction: cardiac complications after stroke. Circ Res 2017;121(4):451–68.

46. Mrozek S, Vardon F, Geeraerts T. Brain temperature: physiology and pathophysiology after brain injury. Anesthesiol Res Pract 2012;2012:1–13.

47. Adatia K, Geocadin RG, Healy R, et al. Effect of body temperature on cerebral autoregulation in acutely comatose neurocritically ill patients. Crit Care Med 2018;46(8):e733.

48. Andrews PJD, Verma V, Healy M, et al. Targeted temperature management in patients with intracerebral haemorrhage, subarachnoid haemorrhage, or acute ischaemic stroke: consensus recommendations. Br J Anaesth 2018;121(4): 768–75.

49. Wrotek SE, Kozak WE, Hess DC, et al. Treatment of fever after stroke: conflicting evidence. Pharmacotherapy 2011;31(11):1085–91.

50. Georgilis K, Plomaritoglou A, Dafni U, et al. Aetiology of fever in patients with acute stroke. J Intern Med 1999;246(2):203–9.

51. Stroke-related pulmonary complications and abnormal respiratory patterns–UpToDate. Available at: https://www.uptodate.com/contents/stroke-related-pulmonary-complications-and-abnormal-respiratory-patterns?search=stroke%20related%20pulmonary%20complications&source=search_result&selectedTitle=1~150&usage_type=default&display_rank=1. Accessed July 15, 2019.

52. CPG_stroke.pdf. Available at: https://www.pedro.org.au/wp-content/uploads/CPG_stroke.pdf. Accessed July 15, 2019.

53. Hocker SE, Tian L, Li G, et al. Indicators of central fever in the neurologic intensive care unit. JAMA Neurol 2013. https://doi.org/10.1001/jamaneurol.2013.4354.

54. McCredie VA, Ferguson ND, Pinto RL, et al. Airway management strategies for brain-injured patients meeting standard criteria to consider extubation. A prospective cohort study. Ann Am Thorac Soc 2017;14(1):85–93.

55. Abu-Snieneh HM, Saleh MYN. Registered nurse's competency to screen dysphagia among stroke patients: literature review. Open Nurs J 2018;12(1):184–94.

56. Lioutas V-A, Hanafy KA, Kumar S. Predictors of extubation success in acute ischemic stroke patients. J Neurol Sci 2016;368:191–4.

57. Chest physiotherapy. Available at: http://currentnursing.com/reviews/chest_physiotherapy.html. Accessed September 17, 2019.

58. Yonaty SA, Schmidt E, El-Zammar Z, et al. Predictors of weaning and extubation failure in mechanically ventilated acute ischemic stroke patients. Gen Med Open 2017;1(2):1–6. https://doi.org/10.15761/GMO.1000110.

59. Karmarkar S, Varshney S. Tracheal extubation. Contin Educ Anaesth Crit Care Pain 2008;8(6):214–20.

60. Bhattacharyya N, Kotz T, Shapiro J. Dysphagia and aspiration with unilateral vocal cord immobility: incidence, characterization, and response to surgical treatment. Ann Otol Rhinol Laryngol 2002;111:672–9.

61. Popat C, Ruthirago D, Shehabeldin M, et al. Outcomes in patients with acute stroke requiring mechanical ventilation: predictors of mortality and successful extubation. Am J Med Sci 2018;356(1):3–9.

62. Bösel J. Use and timing of tracheostomy after severe stroke. Stroke 2017;48(9):2638–43.

63. de J Oliveira I, Da Mota LAN, Freitas SV, et al. Dysphagia screening tools for acute stroke patients available for nurses: a systematic review. Nurs Pract Today 2019;6(3):103–15. https://doi.org/10.18502/npt.v6i3.1253.

64. Shaker R, Geenen JE. Management of dysphagia in stroke patients. Gastroenterol Hepatol 2011;7(5):308–32.

65. Cohen DL, Roffe C, Beavan J, et al. Post-stroke dysphagia: a review and design considerations for future trials. Int J Stroke 2016;11(4):399–411.

66. Shaker R. Rehabilitation of swallowing by exercise in tube-fed patients with pharyngeal dysphagia secondary to abnormal UES opening. Gastroenterology 2002;122:1314–21.

67. Singh S, Hamdy S. Dysphagia in stroke patients. Postgrad Med J 2006;82(968):383–91.

68. Nathadwarawala K, Nicklin J, Wiles C. A timed test of swallowing capacity for neurological patients. J Neurol Neurosurg Psychiatry 1992;55:822–5.

69. Splaingard M, Hutchins B, Sulton L, et al. Aspiration in rehabilitation patients: videofluoroscopy vs bedside clinical assessment. Arch Phys Med Rehabil 1988;69:637–40.

70. Shanahan T, Logemann J, Rademaker A, et al. Chin-down posture effect on aspiration in dysphagic patients. Arch Phys Med Rehabil 1993;74:736–9.

71. Litvan I, Sastry N, Sonies B. Characterizing swallowing abnormalities in progressive supranuclear palsy. Neurology 1997;48:1654–62.

72. Daniels S, Ballo L, Mahoney M, et al. Clinical predictors of dysphagia and aspiration risk: outcome measures in acute stroke patients. Arch Phys Med Rehabil 2000;81:1030–3.

73. Strand E, Miller R, Yorkston K, et al. Management of oral-pharyngeal dysphagia symptoms in amyotrophic lateral sclerosis. Dysphagia 1996;11:129–39.

74. Wirth R, Smoliner C, Jäger M, et al, The DGEM Steering Committee*. Guideline clinical nutrition in patients with stroke. Exp Transl Stroke Med 2013;5(1):14.

75. Joundi RA, Saposnik G, Martino R, et al. Outcomes among patients with direct enteral vs nasogastric tube placement after acute stroke. Neurology 2018;90(7): e544–52.
76. Helldén J, Bergström L, Karlsson S. Experiences of living with persisting post-stroke dysphagia and of dysphagia management–a qualitative study. Int J Qual Stud Health Well-Being 2018;13(sup1):1522194.
77. Chen N, Li Y, Fang J, et al. Risk factors for malnutrition in stroke patients: a meta-analysis. Clin Nutr 2019;38(1):127–35.
78. Collins N, Friedrich L. Nutrition 411: using laboratory data to evaluate nutritional status. Wound Manag Prev 2010;56(3). Available at: https://www.o-wm.com/content/using-laboratory-data-evaluate-nutritional-status.
79. American Heart Association. Stroke may lead to lower vitamin D. 2019. Available at: https://www.heart.org/en/news/2019/08/08/stroke-may-lead-to-lower-vitamin-d. Accessed September 19, 2019.
80. Robbins NM, Swanson RA. Opposing effects of glucose on stroke and reperfusion injury: acidosis, oxidative stress, and energy metabolism. Stroke 2014; 45(6):1881–6.
81. Conrad J, Pawlowski M, Dogan M, et al. Seizures after cerebrovascular events: risk factors and clinical features. Seizure 2013;22(4):275–82.
82. Xu MY. Poststroke seizure: optimising its management. Stroke and Vascular Neurology 2019;4:e000175.
83. Burn J, Dennis M, Bamford J, et al. Epileptic seizures after a first stroke: the Oxfordshire Community Stroke Project. BMJ 1997;315(7122):1582–7.
84. Arboix A, García-Eroles L, Massons JB, et al. Predictive factors of early seizures after acute cerebrovascular disease. Stroke 1997;28(8):1590–4.
85. Labovitz DL, Hauser WA, Sacco RL. Prevalence and predictors of early seizure and status epilepticus after first stroke. Neurology 2001;57(2):200–6.
86. Kilpatrick CJ, Davis SM, Hopper JL, et al. Early seizures after acute stroke. Risk of late seizures. Arch Neurol 1992;49(5):509–11.
87. Shinton RA, Gill JS, Melnick SC, et al. The frequency, characteristics and prognosis of epileptic seizures at the onset of stroke. J Neurol Neurosurg Psychiatry 1988;51(2):273–6.
88. So EL, Annegers JF, Hauser WA, et al. Population-based study of seizure disorders after cerebral infarction. Neurology 1996;46(2):350–5.
89. Lamy C, Domigo V, Semah F, et al. Early and late seizures after cryptogenic ischemic stroke in young adults. Neurology 2003;60(3):400–4.
90. Bladin CF, Alexandrov AV, Bellavance A, et al. Seizures after stroke: a prospective multicenter study. Arch Neurol 2000;57(11):1617–22.
91. Kraus JA, Berlit P. Cerebral embolism and epileptic seizures–the role of the embolic source. Acta Neurol Scand 1998;97(3):154–9.
92. Kilpatrick CJ, Davis SM, Tress BM, et al. Epileptic seizures in acute stroke. Arch Neurol 1990;47(2):157–60.
93. Lo Y-K, Yiu C-H, Hu H-H, et al. Frequency and characteristics of early seizures in Chinese acute stroke. Acta Neurol Scand 1994;90(2):83–5.
94. Berges S, Moulin T, Berger E, et al. Seizures and epilepsy following strokes: recurrence factors. Eur Neurol 2000;43(1):3–8.
95. Reith J, Jørgensen HS, Nakayama H, et al. Seizures in acute stroke: predictors and prognostic significance. The Copenhagen Stroke Study. Stroke 1997;28(8): 1585–9.
96. Lancman ME, Golimstok A, Norscini J, et al. Risk factors for developing seizures after a stroke. Epilepsia 1993;34(1):141–3.

97. Gupta SR, Naheedy MH, Elias D, et al. Postinfarction seizures. A clinical study. Stroke 1988;19(12):1477–81.
98. Cocito L, Favale E, Reni L. Epileptic seizures in cerebral arterial occlusive disease. Stroke 1982;13(2):189–95.
99. Novy J, Logroscino G, Rossetti AO. Refractory status epilepticus: a prospective observational study. Epilepsia 2010;51(2):251–6.
100. Bembenek J, Karlinski M, Kobayashi A, et al. Early stroke-related deep venous thrombosis: risk factors and influence on outcome. J Thromb Thrombolysis 2011;32:96–102.
101. Soroceanu A, Burton DC, Oren JH, et al. Medical complications after adult spinal deformity surgery: incidence, risk factors, and clinical impact. Spine 2016; 41:1718–23.
102. Kelly J, Rudd A, Lewis R, et al. Venous thromboembolism after acute stroke. Stroke 2001;32:262–7.
103. Dizon MAM, De Leon JM. Effectiveness of initiating deep vein thrombosis prophylaxis in patients with stroke: an integrative review. J Neurosci Nurs 2018; 50(5):308–12.
104. Douds GL, Hellkamp AS, Olson DM, et al. Venous thromboembolism in the get with the guidelines-stroke acute ischemic stroke population: incidence and patterns of prophylaxis. J Stroke Cerebrovasc Dis 2014;23:123–9.
105. Li Z, Liu L, Wang Y, et al. Factors impact the adherence rate of prophylaxis for deep venous thrombosis in acute ischemic stroke patients: an analysis of the China National Stroke Registry. Neurol Res 2015;37:427–33.
106. Liu LP, Zheng HG, Wang DZ, et al. Risk assessment of deep-vein thrombosis after acute stroke: a prospective study using clinical factors. CNS Neurosci Ther 2014;20:403–10.
107. American College of Radiology ACR Appropriateness Criteria. Clinical condition: suspected lower-extremity deep vein thrombosis. 2017. Available at: http://acsearch.acr.org/docs/69416/Narrative/2013.
108. Sherman DG, Albers GW, Bladin C, et al. The efficacy and safety of enoxaparin versus unfractionated heparin for the prevention of venous thromboembolism after acute ischaemic stroke (PREVAIL Study): an open-label randomized comparison. Lancet 2007;369:1347–55.
109. Dennis M, Sandercock P, Reid J, et al. Can clinical features distinguish between immobile patients with stroke at high and low risk of deep vein thrombosis? statistical modelling based on the CLOTS trials cohorts. J Neurol Neurosurg Psychiatry 2011;82:1067–73.
110. Kamerkar DR, John MJ, Desai SC, et al. Arrive: a retrospective registry of Indian patients with venous thromboembolism. Indian J Crit Care Med 2016;20:150–8.
111. Powers WJ, Rabinstein AA, Ackerson T, et al. Guidelines for the early management of patients with acute ischemic stroke: 2019 update to the 2018 guidelines for the early management of acute ischemic stroke. Stroke 2019;50.
112. Lansberg MG, O'Donnell MJ, Khatri P, et al. Antithrombotic and thrombolytic therapy for ischemic stroke: antithrombotic therapy and prevention of thrombosis. 9th edition. American College of Chest Physicians evidence-based clinical practice guidelines. Chest 2012;141(2, Suppl):e601S–36S.
113. Morelli VM, Sejrup JK, Småbrekke B, et al. The role of stroke as a trigger for incident venous thromboembolism: results from a population-based. Case-Crossover Study 2019;3(1):e50–7.
114. Theofanidis D, Gibbon B. Nursing interventions in stroke care delivery: an evidence-based clinical review. J Vasc Nurs 2016;34(4):144–51.

115. Smith C, Almallouhi E, Feng W. Urinary tract infection after stroke: a narrative re-view. J Neurol Sci 2019;403:146–52.
116. Yan T, Liu C, Li Y, et al. Prevalence and predictive factors of urinary tract infec-tion among patients with stroke: a meta-analysis. Am J Infect Control 2018; 46(4):402–9.
117. Johnston KC, Li JY, Lyden PD, et al. Medical and neurological complications of ischemic stroke: experience from the RANTTAS trial. RANTTAS investigators. Stroke 1998;29:447–53.
118. Weimar C, Roth MP, Zillessen G, et al. Complications following acute ischemic stroke. Eur Neurol 2002;48:113–40.
119. Hong KS, Kang DW, Koo JS, et al. Impact of neurological and medical compli-cations on 3-month outcomes in acute ischaemic stroke. Eur J Neurol 2008;15: 1324–31.
120. Li J, Yuan M, Liu Y, et al. Incidence of constipation in stroke patients: a system-atic review and meta-analysis. Medicine 2017;96:e7225.
121. Lin CJ, Hung JW, Cho CY, et al. Poststroke constipation in the rehabilitation ward: incidence, clinical course and associated factors. Singapore Med J 2013;54:62409.
122. Whitehead S, Baalbergen E. Post-stroke rehabilitation. S Afr Med J 2019; 109(2):81.
123. American Association of Neuroscience Nurses. Guide to the care of the hospi-talized patient with ischemic stroke. 2nd edition. Glenview (IL): American Asso-ciation of Neuroscience Nurses; 2009.
124. Activase [prescribing information]. South San Francisco (CA): Genentech, Inc; 2018.

# Monitoring for Poststroke Seizures

Cynthia Bautista, PhD, APRN, FNCS, FCNS

## KEYWORDS

- Seizure • Epilepsy • Stroke • Ischemic stroke • Hemorrhagic stroke • Nursing care

## KEY POINTS

- Stroke is the most common cause of secondary epilepsy in adults.
- The incidence of poststroke seizures is higher in intracranial hemorrhage.
- There is limited evidence for the medical management of poststroke seizures.

## INTRODUCTION

Stroke is a major cause of seizure. John Hughlings Jackson recognized the relationship between seizure and stroke over a century ago.[1] The occurrence of poststroke seizure (PSS) is variable and can occur between 2% and 67% of the time.[2,3] Because of the underlying pathologic mechanism, seizures are classified as early onset and late-onset PSS.[4] The probability of a recurrent PSS is as high as 72%.[2] Approximately 30% to 40% of new epilepsy cases among the elderly are accounted for by previous strokes.[5] Poststroke epilepsy can be diagnosed when 2 unprovoked seizures occur after a stroke.[6] Stroke is the most common cause of secondary epilepsy in adults.[7] PSSs are associated with increased mortality, prolonged hospitalizations, and significant disability at discharge.[4,5] The quality of life can be negatively affected when poststroke epilepsy becomes a burden to the stroke survivor.[7]

When a stroke occurs, it will create a lesion to the brain, damaging that area of the cerebral cortex. Scar tissue develops, which will prevent the normal flow of electrical activity of the neurons. A seizure will occur due to the imbalance between excitation and inhibition, causing abnormal neuronal firing. There will be overactivity of excitatory neurotransmitters or underactivity of inhibitory neurotransmitters, which allows for an uncoordinated flow of electrical activity in the brain.

Critical care nurses need to know what the risk factors are, the type of stroke, stroke location, and severity for the poststroke patient who is at risk for an early or late seizure. Nurses should be competent in providing an appropriate seizure assessment and treatment, to provide the best possible outcome for these patients. PSS patients need the critical care nurse to assist them in recovering not only from a stroke but to address concerns for seizure management.

Egan School of Nursing and Health Studies, Fairfield University, 1073 North Benson Road, Fairfield, CT 06824, USA
E-mail address: cabbrain@aol.com

Crit Care Nurs Clin N Am 32 (2020) 85–95
https://doi.org/10.1016/j.cnc.2019.11.006
0899-5885/20/© 2019 Elsevier Inc. All rights reserved.

## TYPES OF SEIZURES
### Focal Seizures

Focal seizures occur in 80% of patients who have seizures.[8] The seizure activity begins in only one part of the cerebral cortex. There are 3 types of focal seizures. Patients with *simple focal seizure* may present with handshaking, "feeling strange," and mouth twitching uncontrollably and are often aware of the event. They may experience aphasia, altered speech, and hallucinations. Often times, there are auras that present before the seizure, with unusual sensations, smells, sounds, or sights; there may even be a feeling of dizziness. A *simple focal seizure* typically lasts up to 90 seconds and may or may not affect consciousness.

Another type of focal seizure is the *complex focal seizure*, which usually lasts about 1 to 2 minutes. It presents with staring straight ahead, looking around, aimless wandering, fidgeting with clothes, facial grimaces, lip-smacking, patting, and rubbing arms (rhythmic twitching) repeatedly. This type of focal seizure tends to have an impaired level of consciousness with confusion, loss of memory, and inability to recall the event.

The last type of focal seizure is the *secondary generalized seizure*, which begins in one part of the brain and spreads to both sides of the brain. The client will first have a focal seizure, which is then followed by a *generalized seizure*.

### Generalized Seizures

Generalized seizures occur in about 20% of people who have seizures.[8] They begin in a widespread fashion that affects both hemispheres of the brain. They tend to have a sudden onset with a loss of consciousness. There are several different types of generalized seizures, including *absence, tonic-clonic, atonic*, and *myoclonic* to name a few.

*Absence seizures*, which were used to be called *petit mal seizures*, have a brief loss of consciousness and some staring or blanking out spells. They may also exhibit rapid blinking, chewing, or aimless movements of the head or limbs. This type of generalized seizure can last between 2 and 15 seconds and is more often found in children.

Another generalized seizure that can occur is a *tonic-clonic seizure*, which was used to be called a *grand mal seizure*. This type of seizure involves the entire cerebral cortex. There are several common signs and symptoms of a generalized seizure, which usually lasts approximately 1 to 2 minutes that the critical care nurse should be able to recognize. Most often, the patient becomes unconscious, not responding to verbal or painful stimulation. Often times they will cry out during the seizure, called an "ictal cry." Muscle jerks or spasms can be seen throughout the ictal phase of a generalized seizure. Incontinence of urine is a common symptom that can occur during a generalized seizure. After the generalized seizure is over, the client does not seem to feel, see, or remember anything that happened during the generalized seizure.

Critical care nurses should be aware that some patients with epilepsy may exhibit strokelike symptoms that can mimic stroke after seizure, called a Todd paralysis. This temporary weakness can last a few seconds up to several hours, most likely due to an exhaustion of the motor cortex neurons. No treatment is necessary except to allow the patient to rest.

## POSTSTROKE SEIZURES

According to the Epilepsy Foundation, PSSs affect 10% of stroke survivors.[9] A seizure can occur within the first 24 hours of a stroke, approximately 3% to 6% of the time.[10] Two to six percent of PSSs will happen in the first 30 days to 12 months after stroke.[4]

Patients with poststroke with a large stroke burden have correlated to a higher risk of PSS.[11] Hemorrhagic strokes are more likely to produce seizures 10% to 16% of the time, whereas an ischemic stroke will produce seizure activity only 2% to 4% of the time.

The following cerebral locations are associated with PSSs, although it is unclear why: parieto-temporal cortex, supramarginal gyrus, and the superior temporal gyrus.[12] PSS are associated with a worse prognosis, for they can increase infarct size and worsen functional recovery.[4]

### Risk Factors

Risk factors that lead to a PSS include intracerebral hemorrhage (ICH), stroke with hemorrhagic transformation, large cortical lesions, and alcohol consumption.[5,13,14] Other risk factors include stroke at a younger age, higher scores on the National Institute of Health Stroke Scale (NIHSS), and having a coagulopathy.[15] The Post-Stroke Epilepsy Risk Scale (PoSERS) (**Table 1**) can be used to predict the risk for poststroke epilepsy.[4] Those patients with acute stroke who have more than 5 items on the PoSERS may be at risk for epilepsy.

### Early Onset Poststroke Seizures

*Early-onset PSSs* can occur within 24 to 48 hours after a stroke[16] and can occur up to 1 week after stroke.[16] Early seizures occur because acute ischemic neuronal injury sets off a cascade of proexcitatory cellular changes, along with membrane depolarization, and lowers the seizure threshold due to a glutamate release and the accumulation of intracellular calcium and sodium.[1,4] Infarct volume size has been correlated with the total duration of depolarizing events. Hyperglycemia at the time of the ischemic event has been suggested to enhance epileptogenesis (gradual process by which a normal brain develops epilepsy).[17] *Early onset seizures* are more likely due to large hemorrhagic strokes. They are also associated with an NIHSS of greater than 14 (0–42). One study found that *early onset PSSs* were more prevalent among male patients.[16] *Early onset seizures* tend to have higher mortality and a prolonged length of stay. There is a 16% chance of PSS recurrence.[18]

The incident rate of seizures after giving alteplase is on the lower side, 4% to 20%.[6] Because of immediate reperfusion, the risk for seizure is decreased for there would be minimal scar tissue. Thrombolytic treatment of patients with ischemic stroke does not prevent *early onset seizures*.[19] Seizures associated with reperfusion syndrome can occur after alteplase has been administered.[7] When perfusion is improved, a cascade of inflammatory responses occurs and contributes to the development of reperfusion

| Table 1 Poststroke epilepsy risk scale | |
|---|---|
| **Item** | **Weight** |
| Supratentorial stroke | 2 |
| Intracerebral hemorrhage involving cortical areas | 2 |
| Seizure occurred 15 d or later after stroke | 2 |
| Ischemia and ongoing neurologic deficit | 1 |
| Stroke caused neurologic deficit with modified Rankin score >3 | 1 |
| Seizure occurred up to 14 d after stroke | 1 |
| Ischemia involving cortical or cortical-subcortical areas | 1 |

syndrome and subsequent seizures.[7] Patients who have received intraarterial thrombectomy are more likely to acquire seizures.[7] This therapy can increase hemorrhagic
transformation rates, leading to possible seizure activity.

### Late-Onset Poststroke Seizures

Late-onset PSSs occur at least 2 weeks and up to 24 months after a stroke.[16] The pathophysiology of PSS activity is the development of scaring of brain tissue (corticomenin-
geal gliosis), altered excitatory neurotransmitter (GABAergic transmission), neural repair
mechanism (axonal sprouting), and effects of iron storage complex (hemosiderin).[4,11]
Late-onset seizures have a recurrence rate of about 50%.[19] Increased stroke disability
and vascular cognitive impairment increase the recurrence of a PSS.[19] These seizures
occur in patients with stroke with a partial anterior circulation syndrome, the presence of
a large cortical infarction located in the parietal-temporal regions.[19]

The estimated risk for a late-onset PSS after ICH is determined by using the CAVE
score.[4,20] The CAVE score is calculated by adding up the points based on the criteria
shown in **Table 2**. The higher the points, the higher the percentage, indicating a more
significant risk for late-onset PSSs after ICH.

### Diagnostic Testing

An electroencephalogram (EEG) should be obtained as soon as possible after the ictal
event. In early onset seizure poststroke patient, 25% have observed periodic lateral-
ized epileptiform discharges (PLEDs).[18] PLEDs are one-sided abnormal electrical activity that is associated with the presence of seizures. A small percentage of
poststroke patients have nonconvulsive status and nonconvulsive status epilepticus.
These types of seizures can lead to unfavorable outcomes. A study by Bentes and colleagues[2] found that 18% of patients with ischemic stroke had interictal (period between seizures) or ictal (during a seizure) epileptiform activity on the EEG during
hospitalization. Most of the ictal activity seen on the EEG occurs in the first 3 days after
stroke. The most frequent finding on EEG is focal slowing (cerebral pathology of the
underlying brain lesion) on the hemispheric side of the infarction.[12] Continuous EEG
monitoring should be considered to capture interictal or ictal abnormalities.[4]

When the critical care nurse looks at the EEG recordings they should note that the x
axis is displaying time and the y axis is displaying voltage. On EEG recordings there
are letters that indicate the lobes of the brain (F-frontal, T-temporal, C-central, P-pa-
rietal, and O-occipital) that the electrodes are positioned over and numbers that represent sides of the brain the electrodes are placed (odd numbers are on the left and even
numbers are on the right). A critical care nurse can look at an EEG recording as they do
an electrocardiogram (ECG). An EEG recording should be reviewed for the following
waveform items:

**Table 2**
**Estimated risk for late-onset poststroke seizures after intracerebral hemorrhage CAVE criteria**

| CAVE | Risk of Late Seizure |
|---|---|
| Cortical involvement of intracerebral hemorrhage (1 point) | 0 point: 0.06% |
| Age <65 (1 point) | 1 point: 3.6% |
| Intracerebral hemorrhage Volume at baseline >10 mL (1 point) | 2 points: 9.8% |
| Early seizure within 7 d of stroke (1 point) | 3 points: 34.8% |
| | 4 points: 46.2% |

- Frequency: increasing or decreasing (number of waves in 1 second)
- Repetition: rhythmic or irregular
- Amplitude: low <20, medium 20 to 50, high >50 μV, isoelectric
- Distribution: focal, lateral, widespread
- Timing: synchronous
- Persistence: paroxysmal or spontaneous
- Morphology—shape of wave
- Symmetry—compare right and left hemispheres

When looking for epileptiform waves (seizure activity), the critical care nurse should see a wave of any duration that has a point peak; they are sharply contoured waveforms. Just as an ECG, an EEG recording can have artifact and the critical care nurse can be very helpful in eliminating this artifact so that an accurate EEG recording can be achieved. Critical care nurses should pay attention to the following to eliminate EEG artifact:

- Bedside equipment interference
- Dried up electrode gel
- Oversedation causing a flat line
- Patient movement
- Eye blinking

Critical care nurses can assist with EEG monitoring by assessing and reporting any changes in the EEG recording to the appropriate health care provider.

To help determine the cause of seizure, a noncontrast head computed tomography can be used in conjunction with clinical and EEG findings. The imaging modality of choice is a brain MRI due to its ability to reveal subtle changes and abnormalities within the brain tissue. Other diagnostic tests that could be considered are blood chemistries, looking for hyponatremia at stroke onset. Hyponatremia can be defined as a serum sodium of less than or equal to 135 mmol/L.[21] This hyponatremia is typically caused by either syndrome of inappropriate antidiuretic hormone (SIADH) or cerebral salt wasting. SIADH is more common than CSW.[22] Hyponatremia has been found to predict PSSs.[23]

## SEIZURE ASSESSMENTS

It is essential to perform a seizure assessment; this will help identify the location of the focus of the seizure. Note that the time of seizure onset and duration of the seizure is necessary information to be assessed. The duration of a seizure will determine if treatment is required. Within 5 minutes of seizure activity, most health care providers will begin treatment, such as administering a benzodiazepine (Lorazepam 1–2 mg intravenously). During the first 5 minutes of a seizure the critical care nurse should observe all that the patient is doing. Airway is always the priority when assessing a patient who is having a seizure. During a seizure, the tongue can obstruct the airway. Assess the oral cavity for secretions, drooling, and bleeding (often due to tongue biting). A decreased level of consciousness is more apt to occur with a generalized seizure. Assess for eye deviation, gaze, and change in pupil size. Eyes will typically deviate in the opposite direction of the seizure activity in the brain. Other body movements occurring during the seizure should be noted. A common motor movement is unilateral hand/arm shaking. Urinary incontinence may also be noted during the seizure.

### Seizure Symptoms Based on Seizure Location

Seizure symptoms will reflect where the location of the seizure occurs in the brain (**Table 3**).[8] Common ipsilateral and contralateral seizure symptoms are shown in **Table 4**.

**Table 3**
**Seizure symptoms based on seizure location**

| Cerebral Lobe | Seizure Symptoms |
|---|---|
| Frontal | • Motor movement, jerking extremity<br>• Movement of head and eyes<br>• Speech arrest, vocal sounds |
| Temporal | • Emotions of fear, sadness, pleasure, flashbacks<br>• Humming, buzzing noises<br>• Feelings of déjà vu<br>• Intense or unpleasant smells or tastes |
| Parietal | • Sensations in one area of the body<br>• Tingling, numbness |
| Occipital | • Flashing lights |

### Ictal (During Seizure) Assessment

During the ictal phase of a seizure, the patient's responsiveness, awareness, language, and motor function should be assessed. Responsiveness can be determined by eliciting a reply or reaction from the patient (Are you having a seizure? What are you feeling right now?). Be sure to continue to assess the patient's orientation to name and location. If the patient cannot respond, continue to assess responsiveness until they are able to respond. Awareness is assessed to determine perception, realization, or knowledge of the situation. Awareness can be evaluated by giving the patient a word or phrase to remember, such as a color or an object, such as a "blue elephant" or "red ball." Language is a systematic means of communicating ideas, and it marks the ability to have an understanding of meanings. Assessment of language by having the patient name an object, such as a pencil or a watch, should be done next. The last part of the ictal assessment is to look at the motor function, which is the ability to use and control muscles and movements. The motor function can be assessed on all extremities by having the patient follow a verbal or demonstrated command such as "stick out your tongue" and "show me two fingers." Continue to assess the patient for head and eye deviation, posturing, and automatisms.

### Postictal (After the Seizure) Assessment

Responsiveness, awareness, motor function, and language should be assessed during the postictal phase. Responsiveness and awareness can be assessed by asking the following questions: Is it over? What just happened? What words did I ask you to remember? (ie, blue elephant). These questions should be repeated until the patient

**Table 4**
**Ipsilateral (one-sided) and contralateral (both sides) common seizure symptoms**

| Common Ipsilateral Symptoms | Common Contralateral Symptoms |
|---|---|
| • Unilateral eye blinking<br>• Automatisms<br>• Periictal headache (temporal lobe)<br>• Last clonic jerk<br>• Postictal nose rubbing | • Arm extension<br>• Postictal paresis (Todd paralysis)<br>• Unilateral clonic activity<br>• Unilateral tonic activity<br>• Unilateral dystonic posturing<br>• Eye deviation<br>• Nystagmus (fast phase) |

can respond. The motor function can be assessed by checking for drift in both the arms and legs, evaluating for a grimace in the face, and if Todd paralysis is present. Language should be assessed next by having the patient name an object (ie, pencil, watch) and asking the question, "What is it used for?"

## NURSING MANAGEMENT
### Ictal Phase (During the Seizure)

The nursing priorities during a seizure are to monitor the airway, stay calm, promote patient safety, and provide reassurance. During a seizure, the patient can be rolled onto one side to prevent aspiration. Nurses should always assist the patient in maintaining their airway by suctioning the oral cavity; teeth may be clenched, hence, do not insert anything into their mouth during this time. Protecting the head from injury may be accomplished by cushioning the patient's head. Assure the patient's bed is in the lowest position and bed rails have been padded. If patient is in a chair, gently lower them to the floor. Clothes should be loosened and eyeglasses removed to provide patient safety. Clearing the area around the patient during a seizure is necessary to protect their body from harm. Be sure not to restrict their body movement. It is crucial to assess all symptoms displayed by the patient during a seizure.

### Postictal Phase (After the Seizure)

The patient should be closely monitored until they are back to their neurologic baseline assessment, usually about 5 to 30 minutes. Critical care nurses should reassure the patient that they are safe. The patient should be assessed for any injury that might have occurred during the seizure. Arms and legs should be assessed for bruises and cuts. After the seizure is over, the critical care nurse should document the event, including a description of seizure activity, level of consciousness, any injuries, and duration of the seizure.

## POSTSTROKE SEIZURE PREVENTATIVE TREATMENT

Practice varies in providing preventative treatment of a PSS, and further research is needed.[14] At this time, there are no clear guidelines or recommendations for PSS prevention. Typically, antiepileptic drug treatment is started when the seizure occurs, rather than preventatively. For the hemorrhagic stroke patient, a prophylactic anticonvulsive may be provided for a short term (7 days).[4] Because of the possible side effects (fatigue, nausea, dizziness) of antiepileptic drugs, prophylactic use may be associated with poorer outcomes.[4]

Critical care nurses should avoid triggers that lower the seizure threshold, such as hypoglycemia, dehydration, sleep deprivation, overexertion, and excessive stress. Excessive alcohol consumption and illicit drug use can also trigger a PSS. Critical care nurses should review with the patient the use of alcohol or illicit drugs (stimulants) before the time of the stroke. Understanding and preventing triggers that can lower the seizure threshold can prevent PSSs.

## POSTSTROKE SEIZURE TREATMENT

Treatment of PSS is managed similar to treating a seizure or epilepsy. After the initial treatment of *early onset seizures*, long-term sustained treatment with antiepileptic drugs is not necessary. Some evidence suggests that antiepileptic drug treatment should begin when the poststroke patient presents with a second or unprovoked recurrent seizure to prevent recurrent seizures.[4] Most of the evidence suggests that anticonvulsant medication should be started after the first *late-onset seizure,* as the recurrence rate is high.[4,19]

The first drugs of choice are levetiracetam (Keppra) or lamotrigine (Lamictal).[19,24] Other common antiepileptic drugs (AEDs) used are phenytoin (Dilantin), carbamazepine (Tegretol), phenobarbital (Solfoton), valproic acid (Depakote), gabapentin (Neurontin), and topiramate (Topamax). Selecting the antiepileptic drug for the poststroke patient would be individualized.

When beginning AED therapy, drug choice should be based on the seizure type. The dose of the AED should be increased to a maximum tolerated dose before changing to another AED. When there is a need to substitute one AED for another, it should be done one drug at a time (monotherapy). There is a 50% chance of failure when starting an AED.[8] Selection of the AED should be based on pharmacokinetics, side effects, dosing, and cost of the AED. When the patient becomes refractory to 2 anticonvulsants, there is an 89% chance of failure, and these patients should be considered for consult to a surgical epilepsy center.[8]

Critical care nurses should be aware of the potential adverse effects AEDs may have on the stroke patient, which will decrease functional outcomes. It has been found that AEDs are associated with poorer stroke outcomes, and they may dampen the brain's neuroplasticity capabilities (ability of the brain to form and reorganize after injury).[10] Levetiracetam (Keppra) can cause irritability and mood disruptions that could interfere with rehabilitation activities. Valproic acid (Depakote) causes fatigue and weight gain, indicating the patient may need more time to recover. Topiramate (Topamax) can slow down cognition, and have word-finding difficulties, which should be assessed, as these may already be stroke deficits the patient may be experiencing. AEDs can affect anticoagulants that many stroke patients are administered to prevent stroke recurrence.[25] Anticoagulants will magnify the effects of AEDs on the liver. PSS patients should be cautioned about their ingestion of alcohol, not only as a risk factor for stroke but also for its harmful effects on the liver. Critical care nurses should discuss the following common reasons for medication nonadherence with their patients: adverse effects, cost, complexity of regimen, cognitive limitations, behavioral issues, lack of education, and denial. The PSS patient needs to understand the importance of compliance regarding their AED regimen in preventing recurrent seizures.[8]

The critical care nurse should discuss possible lifestyle modifications due to PSSs. Daily exercise is beneficial and should be encouraged for PSS patients. Exercise should be monitored and/or done with a buddy. Encourage patients to pace themselves during exercise to avoid hot weather, overdoing, and staying hydrated. PSS patients should be encouraged to have supervision of activities when cooking, swimming, biking, and walking. Safety concerns should be stressed for those patients who are taking AEDs due to gait instability that could lead to risk for falls.

Altering the PSS patient's diet should also be discussed. It is essential to remind the patient to avoid long periods without food and to eat a well-balanced diet. Eating at consistent times of the day is also helpful. They should avoid food and drink that enhance their seizure risk. The PSS patient should consider eliminating sugar and all sweets. The critical care nurse can encourage the patient to try a natural whole foods diet. Consulting with a nutritionist would be beneficial. The critical care nurse should remind the patient that alcohol in small amounts would likely not cause seizure. It is often excessive alcohol use withdrawal that can provoke seizure.

Patients should have the opportunity to discuss with the critical care nurse concerns about social consequences, such as driving and working limitations, and that seizures may affect their poststroke life. For those patients with a current drivers' license, the state agency should be notified of their seizure condition. State agencies of motor vehicles will determine when the patient can resume driving after their most recent seizure. Encourage patients to formally take a driving assessment course after recovery from a stroke. It would be prudent to consider a monitoring device such as a "Life Line" if the patient lives alone or has limiting deficits.

Having seizures can be highly stigmatizing, and educating the patient and family about epilepsy and treatments can help with promoting positive health outcomes.[8] Providing positive feedback about how to manage epilepsy, PSS patients can have their concerns and care needs met. Patients should be referred to an outpatient epileptologist for consult after hospital discharge for brief or continued seizure management.

The European Stroke Organization issued evidence-based guidelines on the management of PSSs and epilepsy.[26] All of the following recommendations and suggestions from this work have a very low quality of evidence and were found to have a weak strength against a strong intervention.[26]

- Because of a low incidence of acute symptomatic seizures poststroke, primary AED prophylaxis is a weak recommendation.
- Because of a low incidence of an acute symptomatic seizure recurrence, there is no need to implement secondary prophylaxis of an AED.
- Because of a low incidence of an unprovoked seizure, there is no need to implement secondary prophylaxis of an AED.
- Because of high seizure recurrence risk, consider secondary AED prophylaxis.
- Because of a low incidence of poststroke unprovoked seizures, there is no need to implement temporary AED treatment.
- There is no consistent evidence to support the use of AEDs to improve functional outcome after stroke; no need to administer AEDs.
- There is insufficient evidence to support the use of temporary treatment with an AED to reduce mortality; no need to administer AEDs.

## OUTCOMES OF POSTSTROKE SEIZURES

Patients with early seizure can have a higher mortality rate at 48 hours poststroke. It is uncertain as to whether or not seizures impair the outcome of an ischemic stroke. Because of the metabolic stress on the vulnerable brain tissue, early seizures might be detrimental.[17] There is a higher mortality rate among stroke patients with seizures after 30 days and 1 year. These patients also encounter poor neurologic scores during acute hospitalization and poor modified Rankin scores (mRS) after discharge. After a late-onset PSS, some patients have experience a worsening stroke sequelae.[17]

## SUMMARY

PSS require special attention and monitoring. Critical care nurses should be aware that seizure assessments are imperative to provide useful information contributing to the diagnosis of seizure type, localization, and lateralization of the seizure focus. Caring for a PSS patient who is having seizures demands the critical care nurse to set priorities and keep the patient safe at all times. Even though there is little evidence in the treatment of PSSs, critical care nurses should advocate for the appropriate treatment to prevent further seizure activities, severe disability, and worse functional outcomes.

## DISCLOSURE

The author has nothing to disclose.

## REFERENCES

1. Jackson J. Epileptiform convulsions from cerebral disease. In: Taylor J, Homes G, Walshe F, editors. Selected writings of John Hughlings Jackson on epilepsy and epileptiform convulsion, vol. 1. London: Hodder and Stoughton Ltd; 1931. p. 330–40.
2. Bentes C, Martins H, Peralta A, et al. Post-stroke seizures are clinically underestimated. J Neurol 2017;264:1978–85.
3. Gilad R. Management of seizures following a stroke. Drugs Aging 2012;29(7): 533–8.
4. Xu M. Poststroke seizure: optimizing its management. Stroke Vasc Neurol 2019;4: e000175.
5. Wang J, Vyas M, Saposnik G, et al. Incidence and management of seizures after ischemic stroke. Neurology 2017;89:1–9.
6. Nesselroth D, Gilad R, Namneh M, et al. Estimation of seizures prevalence in ischemic strokes after thrombolytic therapy. Seizure 2018;62:91–4.
7. Naylor J, Thevathasan A, Churilov L, et al. Association between different acute stroke therapies and development of post stroke seizures. BMC Neurol 2018; 18:61–8.
8. Smith G, Wagner J, Edwards J. Epilepsy update. Am J Nurs 2015;115(6):34–44.
9. Epilepsy foundation. 2019. Available at: https://www.epilepsy.com/article/2018/5/post-stroke-seizures-and-epilepsy-frequently-asked-questions/. Accessed July 27, 2019.
10. American Stroke Association 2019. Available at: https://www.strokeassociation.org/en/about-stroke/effects-of-stroke/physical-effects-of-stroke/physical-impact/controlling-post-stroke-seizures/. Accessed July 27, 2019.
11. Stefanidou M, Das R, Beiser A, et al. Incidence of seizures following initial ischemic stroke in a community-based cohort. Seizure 2017;47:105–10.
12. Pitkanen A, Roivanen R, Lukasiuk K. Development of epilepsy after ischaemic stroke. Lancet Neurol 2016;15:185–97.
13. Zhang C, Wang X, Wang Y, et al. Risk factors for post-stroke seizures: a systematic review and meta-analysis. Epilepsy Res 2014;108:1806–16.
14. Leung T, Leung H, Soo YO, et al. The prognosis of acute symptomatic seizures after ischaemic stroke. J Neurol Neurosurg Psychiatry 2017;88(1):86–94.
15. Conrad J, Pawlowski M, Dogan M, et al. Seizures after cerebrovascular events: risk factors and clinical features. Seizure 2013;22:275–82.
16. Qazi T, Siddiqui A, Lakhair M, et al. Frequency of early seizures in patients of acute ischemic stroke. J Liaquat Uni Med Health Sci 2016;15(3):143–6.
17. Camilo O, Goldstein L. Seizures and epilepsy after ischemic stroke. Stroke 2004; 35:1769–75.
18. De Reuck J. Management of stroke-related seizures. Eur Neurol Rev 2007; 2:55–6.
19. De Reuck J. Seizures and epilepsy related to stroke. EC Neurology 2019;11(4): 202–3.
20. Haapaniemi E, Strbian D, Rossi C, et al. The CAVE score for predicting late seizures after intracerebral hemorrhage. Stroke 2014;45:1971–6.
21. Ehtesham M, Mohmand M, Raj K, et al. Clinical spectrum of hyponatremia in patients with stroke. Cureus 2019;11(8):e5310.
22. Saleem S, Yousuf I, Gul A, et al. Hyponatremia in stroke. Ann Indian Acad Neurol 2014;17:55–7.

23. Wang G, Jia H, Chen C, et al. Analysis of risk factors for first seizure after stroke in Chinese patients. Biomed Res Int 2013. https://doi.org/10.1155/2013/702871.

24. Huang Y, Chi N, Kuan Y, et al. Efficacy of phenytoin, valproic acid, carbamaze-pine and new antiepileptic drugs on control of late-onset post-stroke epilepsy in Taiwan. Eur J Neurol 2015;22:1459–68.

25. Kim B, Sila C. Seizures in ischemic stroke. In: Koubeissi M, et al, editors. Seizures in cerebrovascular disorders. New York: Springer; 2015. p. 17–29.

26. Holtkamp M, Beghi E, Benninger F, et al. European stroke organization guidelines for the management of post-stroke seizures and epilepsy. Eur Stroke J 2017;2(2):103–15.

# Stroke Rehabilitation

Maureen Le Danseur, MSN, CNS, ACNS-BC, CRRN, CCM

## KEYWORDS

- Stroke rehabilitation • Rehabilitation nursing • Functional abilities

## KEY POINTS

- To outline the admission criteria for acute inpatient rehabilitation.
- To expand understanding of the rehabilitation nurses role in stroke recovery.
- To highlight the importance of the interdisciplinary team approach.
- Discuss the psychosocial aspects of post-stroke care.

## INTRODUCTION

Approximately 795,000 people experience a stroke annually, and 60%, or approximately 465,000 of those require some type of rehabilitation.[1] Not all strokes are created equal, they are as unique as the patients who experience them. During the acute hospitalization, families are searching for predictive signs of recovery, and as nurses we want to provide them that support. Unfortunately, it is not often plausible to predict the recovery trajectory that any stroke patient will take. What we do know is that, with timely interventions, we are seeing improved outcomes,[2] although complete recovery may not be possible. The rehabilitation goal is to improve quality of life, attaining independence, along with facilitating and encouraging family and community participation.

## REHABILITATION ADMISSION CRITERIA

The Centers for Medicare and Medicaid Services (CMS) criteria for admission to an inpatient rehabilitation facility (IRF)[3] include the following:

- The patient must require active and ongoing therapeutic intervention from multiple disciplines, which can include physical therapy (PT), occupational therapy (OT), speech language pathology (SLP), and orthotics/prosthetics. One of these disciplines must be PT or OT.
- Patients must require and be able to participate in an intense rehabilitation program. This includes 3 hours of therapy per day for at least 5 days per week, starting on the day of admission.

Sharp Memorial Rehabilitation Center, 2999 Health Center Drive, San Diego, CA 92123, USA
E-mail address: maureen.ledanseur@sharp.com

Crit Care Nurs Clin N Am 32 (2020) 97–108
https://doi.org/10.1016/j.cnc.2019.11.004
0899-5885/20/© 2019 Elsevier Inc. All rights reserved.

- There must be a reasonable expectation that they will make measurable improvements due to the program. For this to occur, the patient must be medically stable.
- Patients require physician oversight from a rehabilitation physician to assess their physical and rehabilitation needs.
- Patients require a coordinated interdisciplinary approach to rehabilitation.

Inpatient rehabilitation criteria is strict and often the reason patients are not accepted. Though after a stay at a skilled nursing facility (SNF) or a long-term acute care facility (LTAC), with improvement in their clinical status they may be escalated to an IRF when appropriate.

## THE DIAGNOSIS

Your stroke patient is now ready for transfer to an IFR and you are calling to give report. Never underestimate the value of a detailed diagnosis during both the acute and rehabilitation phase. Knowing whether the patient had a right versus left hemispheric stroke and a detailed description of their deficits can prove very valuable, giving the rehabilitation nurse a snapshot of what to expect (**Table 1**).

The rehabilitation nurse will have experience correlating the brain injury as a result of a stroke and associated deficits along with what to expect with regards to function and behavior. The cerebral vessel(s) occluded and subsequent area of infarct will give a more complete understanding of the clinical symptom manifestations the nurse would expect to see.[4]

Behaviorally, a patient with a left-sided stroke demonstrates an awareness of their deficits, tends to be slow or cautious with tasks, and can be easily frustrated. Patients with a right-sided stroke demonstrate distracted and impulsive behavior, poor memory, and diminished concentration.

## SCENARIO

- 59 M transferred to a rehabilitation unit after a right middle cerebral artery (RMCA) stroke. He was noted lethargic (sleepy), requiring the team to wake him to eat, turn, and participate in therapies.
- He was dysphasic (difficulty swallowing), and had difficulty maintaining his oral secretions. A modified barium swallow revealed a moderate risk for aspiration.

**Table 1**
**Left versus right hemispheric strokes**

| Left Hemispheric Strokes | Right Hemispheric Strokes |
| --- | --- |
| Language deficits—expressive or receptive | Visual and spatial deficits |
| Right hemiplegia or hemiparesis | Left hemiplegia or hemiparesis |
| Confuses L and R | Gets lost, misjudges distance |
| Difficulty reading or writing | Distorted body image |
| Aware of deficits, easily frustrated | Poor judgment, unrealistic thoughts |
| Tends to be slow and cautious | Poor memory and concentration |
| Right homonymous hemianopia | Left homonymous hemianopia |
| (see glossary of terms) | (see glossary of terms) |
| | Quick and impulsive (needs supervision) |
| | Distractible |

Data from Lehman C, Association of Rehabilitation Nurses. The specialty practice of rehabilitation nursing: a core curriculum. Association of Rehabilitation Nurses, 2015, pp 471-510.

He was placed on a pureed diet with moderately thickened liquids, and required supervision at meal time. A nursing assistant, nurse, or speech therapist can provide this supervision.

- He was demonstrating dysarthria (slurred speech), compromising his ability to communicate. A language board was implemented to assist with communicating his basic needs. There were pictures of a plate, drinking glass, toilet, bed with side rails, nurse, wheelchair, toothbrush, eyeglasses, stop sign, and the words yes and no. This allowed him to point to the item that best communicated his need or response. He was able to answer yes and no questions with 90% accuracy, which was another tool used to improve communication.
- Signs of a left-sided visual field deficit were evident. When he received his meal, he only ate items on the right side of the tray. This prompted the team to guide him to turn his head, and to scan his environment while eating and ambulating. This measure significantly improved his safety and awareness. A move to a different room where the layout had his family sitting on his left side during their visits increased his need to continue scanning to the left.
- He was also experiencing bladder incontinence, this was not a problem before his stroke. A timed voiding program was initiated. Patients are toileted every 2 hours during the day and every 4 hours at night. This continuity helps to retrain the brain to respond to bladder fullness by going to the restroom.[5]

As he improved and became more alert, he began to exhibit impulsive behavior. This behavior included getting out of bed without calling for assistance, setting off his bed alarm, and attempting to remove his wheelchair seat belt, all actions making him at higher risk for falls. The nursing plan of care included problems addressing swallow, communication, fall risk, and bladder incontinence.

## REHABILITATION NURSING

Rehabilitation is "the process of helping a person who has suffered an illness or injury restore lost skills and regain maximum self-sufficiency."[6] The rehabilitation nurse is an essential member part of the coordinated interdisciplinary team, assisting patients and families to develop an altered lifestyle within a safe environment. The rehabilitation nursing specialty requires a focus on goals, outcomes, the attainment or maintenance of functional capacity, the ability to understand long-range patient needs, and a focus on wellness.

"A person with a disability has intrinsic values that transcend the disability; each person is a unique holistic being who has the right and responsibility to make informed personal choices regarding health and lifestyle."[7] The Self-Care Deficit Theory by Dorothy Orem is based on the premise that it is the responsibility of the rehabilitation nurse to assist patients in compensating for and overcoming their deficits. Functioning independently helps us to preserve and foster self-esteem. This theory is part of the foundation of rehabilitation nursing.[8]

Sam experienced a left hemispheric stroke, leaving him with a right hemiplegia and aphasia. One morning, Sam was talking on the phone with his family. The occupational therapist had placed a strap over the receiver of his landline phone to assist him with picking up, holding, and hanging up the phone. As the rehabilitation nurse appeared, Sam decided to terminate the call. After doing so, he attempted to hang up the phone but missed the phone base. He tried again but was unsuccessful. At this point, he looked at the rehabilitation nurse and said, "Aren't you going to help me?" To which she replied, "I know you would like me to help you with this, but you are here to relearn how to do these types of tasks. Will you try it again?" He did. As the receiver dropped into the cradle, his face lit up. He was so proud of his accomplishment. It was another step toward self-care independence. As the rehabilitation nurse, it would have been easy to replace the receiver for him, but that would have denied him this victory. This is rehabilitation nursing.

## GOAL SETTING

Upon admission, with the help of physical medicine and rehabilitation (PM&R) physician, in collaboration with PT, OT, SLP, neuropsychology, and the rehabilitation nurse, a comprehensive assessment of the patient's deficits and subsequent challenges is documented. The next step is to create a person-centered plan of care, so that patients, families, and staff agree on the same goals of care. This measure facilitates a mutual understanding of the plan and an increased willingness on the part of the patient to participate.

## REHABILITATION NURSING FOCUS
### Skin Assessment

Implementing strategies to keep skin intact, heal current wounds, and alleviate pressure areas is a priority. Educational opportunities involving patients and families while turning the patient in bed, transitioning in and out of a wheelchair, and how to perform a skin assessment at home are used.

### Goal
To prevent pressure ulcer formation during their hospital stay and provide education to the patient and family to encourage habitual position changes for skin protection at home.[5]

### Bladder Incontinence

Post-stroke patients will fall into 1 of the following 3 categories. Some will never experience incontinence, some will experience incontinence and will not be able to regain continence, and the majority are incontinent at first, but with retraining are able to become continent again. Timed voiding is used to retrain their brain to recognize the sensation to void and the appropriate response of going to the restroom.[5] Performing a urinary history will assist you in determining if complete continence is feasible. If a 70-year-old woman has a history of urinary urge and stress incontinence for 15 years, the goal should be to return her to her prestroke continence level. Diapers or adult briefs are used for patients experiencing incontinence.

### Goal
Help return the patient to bladder continence or teach the family how to manage incontinence at home.

### Bowel

Post-stroke patients will fall into categories similar to bladder. The majority of stroke patients will regain continence with retraining; however, for some bowel continence may not be possible. Retraining involves timed toileting using their prestroke bowel patterns. Often time's patients present to rehabilitation who have not had a bowel movement in several days. The initial challenge is to get their bowels moving again. As the intensive or acute care nurse, you can help by letting the provider know each day that the patient has or has not had a bowel movement. Providers tend to have their own preferred medications for constipation. Use of standing and as-needed laxatives and stool softeners should be incorporated into the daily bowel regimen if indicated.

### Goal

To facilitate the return of continence, retrain patients in bowel control, and limit incontinent episodes.

### Pain

Pain assessment will help to drive a successful plan of care. There are patients who do not have complaints of pain after stroke. Others may find the rehabilitation process causes discomfort owing to increased activity, overuse of the intact side of their body, and muscle spasms. Pain caused by preexisting comorbidities such, as arthritis, gout, or chronic back pain, may also be an issue.[5]

After a stroke, shoulder subluxation can occur. This is a partial dislocation of the shoulder joint caused by the weakened supraspinatus and deltoid muscles. This condition in and of itself is not usually painful, but our manipulation and improper positioning of the joint can cause pain. The primary intervention used to alleviate this pain should be supporting the shoulder, proper positioning, using a lapboard when sitting in a wheelchair, and range of motion exercises.[5,9]

Two years ago, all of our patients were using some type of opioid for pain relief. Today, the majority of our stroke patients are finding that acetaminophen is adequate, especially if they use it in conjunction with some nonpharmacologic modalities.

Nonpharmacologic pain modalities for the stroke population might include:

- *Positioning*—decrease muscle spasms and relieve pressure
- *Meditation*—engaging in reflection and controlled breathing with a focus on relaxation of mind and body
- *Music therapy*—used to decrease stress and anxiety[10]
- *Reiki*—a gentle hands-on technique that harmonizes a person's life force[11]
- *Hand massage*—to stimulate nerves, increase blood flow, and decrease stress
- *Aromatherapy*—using essential oils or scents to increase relaxation can be beneficial (use caution because people with fragrance sensitivities may have a reaction if they are in the immediate vicinity)
- *Pet therapy*—a pet visit by a certified therapy pet is used to reduce stress[12] (family pets may visit, but need to remain outside unless they are an Emotional Support Animal)

### Goal

Control pain to enhance participation in rehabilitation therapies and if possible avoid or limit narcotic use.

### Hydration, Nutrition, and Swallowing

Nutrition and hydration are the foundation building blocks for post-stroke recovery. There is a risk for malnutrition, dehydration and weight loss due to dysphagia, depression and perceptual deficits. There is a risk for malnutrition, dehydration and weight loss. This affects 35% to 50% of post-stroke patients and is an indicator of poor outcome.[5] After a modified barium swallow, modified texture meals may be required and swallow strategies implemented. This may include 100% supervision during a meal by nursing, turning head toward the weaker side before swallowing in an attempt to decrease aspiration risk, chin tuck, small bites, small sips, and/or no straws. Based on their assessment, the SLP will determine the need for precautions and communicate recommendations with the nursing team.

If mildly or moderately thickened liquids are ordered, consider using a gum-containing thickener over a starch-based thickener. The reason for this is, that over time, the starch-based products become significantly thinner (increasing aspiration risk) compared with the gum-based drink.[13] Many patients find it difficult to drink something with a thickened consistency, and therefore limits their fluid intake. This is where working with the rehabilitation team, including the family, to encourage intake becomes important.

### Goal
Prevent aspiration and provide adequate nutrition measured by percentage eaten or calorie count and hydration demonstrated by adequate fluid intake.

### Communication

With certain types of stroke, communication deficits can be very challenging. SLP will identify barriers and potential solutions to opening lines of communication between the rehabilitation team and patient. Tools often used are:

- An interpreter if there is a language barrier
- Ensure the patient has eyeglasses and hearing aids used before the stroke
- Communication boards allow the patient to point to a picture to communicate their needs
- Some patients can speak but they need time to form and articulate words, it is prudent to give them time to comprehend and respond
- Minimize background noise, get patient's attention, and use simple statements to communicate when receptive (understanding) aphasia is present
- Educating the family to use these interventions will improve patient and family satisfaction

### Goals
Assist the patient in improving their communication abilities. Minimize patient frustration related to their inability to communicate clearly. Arrange outpatient or home health SLP as needed at discharge.

| Table 2 Glossary of terms | | |
|---|---|---|
| **Terms** | **Meaning** | **Treatment/Team Members** |
| Acalculia | Inability to perform basic math skills following a stroke | Speech therapy |
| Apraxia | Problem finding words or inability to remember the steps in a task such as brushing hair | Speech therapy or OT |
| Ataxia | Lack of coordination of voluntary movement | Any or all of the therapists depending on affected area |
| Broca's aphasia (expressive aphasia) | Partial loss of ability to produce language but understanding language is intact | Speech therapy May need communication board to express basic needs |
| | | *(continued on next page)* |

**Table 2**
*(continued)*

| Terms | Meaning | Treatment/Team Members |
| --- | --- | --- |
| Dysarthria | Trouble forming words, slurred or slow speech | Speech therapy |
| Dysgraphia | Trouble writing | Speech therapy |
| Dyslexia | Trouble reading | Speech therapy |
| Dysphagia | Inability to swallow safely; aspiration risk | Swallow study, modified barium swallow, speech therapy |
| Hemiplegia | Muscle weakness on one side, may include numbness | Physical therapy or OT, proper positioning |
| Homonymous hemianopsia | Visual field loss in the same side of both eyes | Usually resolves on its own or may need neuro-ophthalmology<br>Use scanning technique to help patient see the whole picture |
| Jargon | Speech incomprehensible but seems to make sense to patient | Speech therapy |
| Labile emotions | Exaggerated changes in mood that can even be inappropriate | Distraction can be helpful, introduce an activity<br>Awareness of what is happening |
| Memory changes | Affects short-term memory more than long term | Speech therapy, use of memory books, timers on a phone or watch can be helpful |
| Neglect | To totally ignore 1 side of their body, the room, a page, or their meal tray | Speech will teach patient to scan to the neglected side<br>Nursing will provide reminders |
| Perseveration | Keeps repeating the same phrase or word | The team uses distraction by starting a new conversation<br>Educate family |
| Uninhibited bladder | A disconnect between the sense to void and knowing when and how to use the restroom | Nursing will use timed voiding will help to reestablish this connection and usually correct the incontinence |
| Uninhibited bowel | A disconnect between the sense to empty bowel and knowing when and how to use the restroom | Nursing will use timed voiding will help to reestablish this connection and usually correct the incontinence |
| Wernicke's aphasia (receptive aphasia) | Will have trouble understanding what is being said or written | Speech therapy |

## Fall Risk

The fall rate for stroke patients during the rehabilitative phase of care can be as low as 10% or as high as 47%.[14] Falls can occur with nursing or with the therapist during a therapy session. Some common causes are knee buckling during ambulation, forgetting to call for help owing to poor memory, they had a good therapy session and are sure they can go to the bathroom independently, impulsivity, or medication side effects. Fall prevention strategies used include, bed and wheelchair alarms, pelvic restraints, bed enclosures, and a sitter as needed. High-risk patients are placed close to the nurse's station, rooms are kept clutter free, and family members may spend the night. Staying with the patient during toileting is recommended owing to the high risk for falls. Attempts are made to turn away to provide privacy while toileting, although one hand must be on the patient's shoulder for safety.[5]

### Goals

Fall and injury prevention. Educating patients and families on fall prevention strategies that can be used during the IRF stay and at home.

## AN INTERPROFESSIONAL APPROACH: "IT TAKES A VILLAGE"

An interdisciplinary team dynamic is essential to the successful rehabilitation patient experience. Each member of the team brings his or her own expertise and is aware that success necessitates working together toward common goal completion. The rehabilitation interdisciplinary team is required to meet weekly to discuss each patient's plan of care. The Commission on Accreditation of Rehabilitation Facilities (CARF) recommends that patients and families participate in this process. These meetings facilitate the dissemination of current information; helps remove barriers, celebrates progress, and facilitates discharge planning.

Rehabilitation centers use the Functional Independence Measures (FIM)[15,16] to quantify patient's progress and outcomes. The following 18 items—eating, grooming, bathing, upper body dressing, lower body dressing, toileting, bladder management, bowel management, bed to chair transfer, toilet transfer, shower transfer, locomotion, stairs, cognitive comprehension, expression, social interaction, problem solving, and memory—are scored from 1 to 7 to indicate the patient's level of assistance needed.

- 1 = total assistance (staff assist 100%)
- 2 = Maximum assistance (patient does 25% and staff assist with 75%)
- 3 = Moderate assistance (patient does 50% and staff assist with 50%)
- 4 = Minimal assistance (patient does 75% and staff assist with 25%)
- 5 = Set up with no physical contact (staff gathers equipment or opens containers)
- 6 = Modified independence (patient independent but uses equipment)
- 7 = Independent

Uniform Data System (UDS) collect this data from rehabilitation facilities around the country. This enables rehabilitation facilities to benchmark and compare gains with other similar rehabilitation centers. Beginning October 1, 2019, FIM scoring will no longer be used to determine the Case Mix Grouping, which is similar to a diagnosis-related group (DRG) used in the acute care setting and determines the patient's approved length of stay. CMS is transitioning Rehabilitation Facilities to the Standardized Patient Assessment Data Elements (SPADE) tool. SPADE will be completed by rehabilitation centers, skilled nursing facilities, long-term acute care centers, and home health agencies to facilitate standardization of information being reported to

CMS. SPADE will classify level of assistance, but the definitions will be different and the items covered expanded.

## REHABILITATION = RELEARNING

On admission, the rehabilitation team completes an assessment of patient and families readiness to learn. Nationally, the average length of stay in an IRF for stroke patients is 15 days. Relearning will include activities of daily living; bed, wheelchair, and car transfers; walking alone or with a device; communicating; swallowing; problem solving; bladder and bowel control; pressure reliefs; blood pressure control; stroke prevention; medication administration; and fall prevention, just to name a few. Almost every nursing and therapy contact should include education.

## NEUROPSYCHOLOGY

A specialist used primarily in the rehabilitation setting is the neuropsychologist. Neuropsychologists study the relationship between behavior, emotions, cognition, and brain function. They individualize stroke education, helping the patient and family to understand what their challenges might be, taking into account their stroke type and location. They also perform testing for various purposes, including the ability to return to work. They work with staff on behavior management plans and provide emotional support for patients and staff throughout the rehabilitation process.

## EMOTIONAL SUPPORT

Once patients are medically stable and recognize life will be different, their coping skills are tested. There are many unknowns. Will I be able to go back to work? Will I be able to communicate? Will I be able to climb the stairs to get into my house? How will my friends and family see me now? How do I adjust to my new self-image?

Listening to the patient's story and allowing them to grieve is important, helping them to work through how different their life is now, hoping for the best but dealing with the present. The team works to decrease stress by allowing the patient and family to have control over their care choices. The nurse, neuropsychologist, social worker, and chaplain all play an important role in this process.[5,17]

## FAMILY AND CAREGIVERS

The rehabilitation goal is to enable patients to return home upon discharge. This will involve family and/or caregiver support. Strokes have the most impact on the patient, but also have significant life-altering effects on the family. The family member is now transitioning into the role of caregiver and may need to learn other roles as well. For this reason, all rehabilitation patients and their families interact with a social worker.

The social worker is available for providing community resources, support groups, help caregivers to tap into unrecognized resources such as friends, neighbors, church groups, and family for help and respite. The social worker is an integral part of the discharge process, working with case management to set a plan in motion as early as possible during the IRF stay. The social worker will assess for available community resources, educate caregivers in the importance of self-care, arrange for department of motor vehicles (DMV) handicap parking, disability paperwork completion, and assist with identifying other medical insurance resources that might be available.

Engaging family members or caregivers early in the rehabilitation process is vital. The team can assist with teaching the patient and caregivers coping skills. Helping them to learn from both positive and negative experiences associated with caregiving. Due to the high risk of post-stroke depression, supporting the patient and family's ability to problem solve will potentially translate into an improved quality of life.[18,19]

## SEXUAL FUNCTIONING AFTER A STROKE

Recent research shows that couples want information about their future sexual relationships.[5,20] Occasionally, patients are curious and may ask questions about sex early in their rehabilitation stay, whereas others want to know but are too embarrassed to ask. We have integrated this education into our process for all patient who are open to receive it.

There are multiple factors that will affect their sexual abilities moving forward. Sensation will affect their erogenous zones. Mobility will affect their ability to sustain certain positions during sex. The ability to communicate can interfere with picking up your partners subtle cues that they are interested in engaging in sex. Initially, fatigue can become a large barrier. Medications for blood pressure, depression, and seizures can cause erectile dysfunction. What should they do if this occurs? When is it safe to start having sex again? Will having sex cause another stroke? If you had a stroke, would you like to have the answers to these questions?

## COMMUNITY REENTRY

A part of any rehabilitation program should include working with a recreational therapists, who engages with patients and encourages them to return to their previous hobbies or activities. By incorporating their previous recreational activities into their rehab program, creates an opportunity for them to practice their therapy in a fun and enjoyable way. A recent study evaluated 24 participants in an art-based creative engagement experience. The findings showed that the patients fell into 1 of 4 categories: they had an appreciation of the opportunity, an appreciation of self, an appreciation of others, or a renewed appreciation of life, all of which were beneficial.[21]

Available activities can include card games, art class, music, knitting, crocheting, yoga classes, gardening, golf, and interactions with pets. Opportunities to take each patient on an outing prior to discharge, such as to a restaurant, shopping excursion, movie or fishing can be beneficial. This allows them to adjust to being in public and helps them start to adjust to different responses to their new body, changes to their mobility, or communication abilities.

## DRIVING

"In approximately 30% of stroke survivors, it is clear from the onset that driving will no longer be possible. Approximately 33% of survivors will be able to return to driving with little or no retraining, and 35% will require driving-related rehabilitation before they can resume safe driving again."[22] At the time of discharge, patients are usually instructed not to drive initially. The topic is then discussed between patient and physician in the outpatient setting. Some rehabilitation centers have driving simulation programs that address motor, visual, cognitive and perceptive skills. Once cleared by OT they would be able to retest at the DMV if required by their state.

## SUMMARY

Your patients have survived thanks to you, but they still have a challenging journey ahead. Ultimately, all short-term goals will lead to successful long-term goal achievements and a safe transition home. Upon discharge, referrals are made to either outpatient or home health services, to continue the rehabilitation process. Rehabilitation should begin the moment health care is initiated, to incorporate wellness and self-reliance into their care. "A major goal in educating all health care providers is to prepare them to 'think rehab' from the moment of initial contact with the stroke patient."[7] We are all part of the rehabilitation process, a link in the chain toward improved quality of life.

## STROKE REHABILITATION TERMINOLOGY

**Table 2** lists terms commonly used by the rehabilitation team.[5]

## DISCLOSURE

The author has nothing to disclose.

## REFERENCES

1. Available at: https://www.cdc.gov/stroke/facts.htm. Accessed August 12, 2019.
2. Brandstater ME, Shutter LA. Rehabilitation interventions during acute care of stroke patients. Top Stroke Rehabil 2002;9(2):48–56.
3. Available at: https://www.cms.gov/Outreach-and-Education/Medicare-Learning-Network-MLN/MLNMattersArticles/Downloads/SE17036.pdf. Accessed September 20, 2019.
4. Tocco S. Identify the vessel, recognize the stroke. Am Nurse Today 2011; 6(9):8–11.
5. Lehman C, Association of Rehabilitation Nurses. The specialty practice of rehabilitation nursing: a core curriculum. Chicago: Association of Rehabilitation Nurses; 2015. p. 471–510.
6. Shiel W. Definition of rehabilitation. Orange, CA: Medicine Net; 2018.
7. Hickey J. The clinical practice of neurological and neurosurgical nursing. Philadelphia, PA: Lippincott Williams & Wilkins; 2014. p. 511–39.
8. Biggs A. Orem's self-care deficit nursing theory: update on the state of the art and science. Nurs Sci Q 2019;21(3):200–6.
9. Lindgren I, Jönsson AC, Norrving B, et al. Shoulder pain after stroke: a prospective population-based study. Stroke 2007;38(2):343–8.
10. Le Danseur M, Crow AD, Stutzman SE, et al. Music as a therapy to alleviate anxiety during inpatient rehabilitation for stroke. Rehabil Nurs 2019;44(1):29–34.
11. Birocco N, Guillame C, Storto S, et al. The effects of reiki therapy on pain and anxiety in patients attending a day oncology and infusion services unit. Am J Hosp Palliat Care 2012;29(4):290–4.
12. Burres S, Edwards NE, Beck AM, et al. Incorporating pets into acute inpatient rehabilitation: a case study. Rehabil Nurs 2016;41(6):336–41.
13. Killeen L, Lansink M, Schröder D. Tolerability and product properties of a gum-containing thickener in patients with dysphagia. Rehabil Nurs 2018;43(3):149–57.
14. Weerdesteyn V, de Niet M, van Duijnhoven HJ, et al. Falls in individuals with stroke. J Rehabil Res Dev 2008;45(8):1195–213.
15. Available at: https://www.udsmr.org/Documents/The_FIM_Instrument_Background_Structure_and_Usefulness.pdf. Accessed September 20, 2019.
16. Linacre J, Heinemann AW, Wright BD, et al. The structure and stability of the functional independence measure. Arch Phys Med Rehabil 1994;75(2):127–32.

17. Sailus MC. The role of the chaplain in the interdisciplinary care of the rehabilitation patient. Rehabil Nurs 2017;42(2):90–6.

18. Robinson-Smith G, Harmer C, Sheeran R, et al. "Couples' coping after stroke-a pilot intervention study. Rehabil Nurs 2015;41(4):218–29.

19. Ren H, Liu C, Li J, et al. Self-perceived burden in the young and middle-aged inpatients with stroke: a cross-sectional survey. Rehabil Nurs 2016;41(2):101–11.

20. Krautz DD, Van Horn ER. Sex and intimacy after stroke. Rehabil Nurs 2017;42(6):333–40.

21. Sit JWH, Chan AWH, So WKW, et al. Promoting holistic well-being in chronic stroke patients through leisure art-based creative engagement. Rehabil Nurs 2017;42(2):58–66.

22. Akinwuntan AE, Wachtel J, Rosen PN. Driving simulation for evaluation and rehabilitation of driving after stroke. J Stroke Cerebrovasc Dis 2012;21(6):478–86.

# What Is Stroke Certification and Does It Matter?

Linda M. Bresette, DNP, MSN, NP-C

## KEYWORDS

- Stroke certification • Stroke systems of care • Primary stroke center
- Comprehensive stroke center • Benefits of certification

## KEY POINTS

- Stroke care and treatment have undergone rapid transformation over the past 2 decades.
- These developments in treatment have necessitated rapid identification of stroke symptoms and hierarchal levels of stroke systems of care.
- Certification of stroke centers is provided by several different agencies and can be costly and is often perceived as burdensome.
- Certification includes the following benefits: provides an objective assessment of stroke care, creates a cohesive team, recognizes the nurse's contribution, and improves patient outcomes.
- The intensive care unit nurse is critical to an organization successfully obtaining stroke center certification. Both patients and nurses benefit from stroke center certification and quality improvement programs.

## BACKGROUND

An acute stroke is a medical emergency with treatments that are time dependent. Stroke care has undergone tremendous transformation over the past 2 decades. For ischemic strokes, the introduction of intravenous thrombolysis (alteplase) and endovascular therapies such as mechanical thrombectomy have been imperative to reducing disability and death from stroke[1]

Recombinant tissue plasminogen activator (alteplase) was approved by the US Food and Drug Administration in 1996 for use within 3 hours of onset of stroke symptoms. In 2008, the time window for intravenous (IV) alteplase was extended to 4.5 hours after symptom onset as a result of the European Cooperative Acute Stroke Study trial that tested the efficacy and safety of alteplase administered between 3.0 and 4.5 hours after the onset of a stroke[2] A recent trial by Ma and colleagues[3] reviewed the possibility of extending the alteplase window even further to 9 hours in select patients.

Updated guidelines from the American Heart Association/American Stroke Association (AHA/ASA) in 2015 expanded the window of treatment for thrombectomy from

Comprehensive Stroke Program, Neurology, Brigham and Women's Hospital, Boston, MA, USA
*E-mail address:* lbresette@bwh.harvard.edu

Crit Care Nurs Clin N Am 32 (2020) 109–119
https://doi.org/10.1016/j.cnc.2019.11.002
0899-5885/20/© 2019 Elsevier Inc. All rights reserved.

ccnursing.theclinics.com

6 hours to 16 to 24 hours after last seen well.[4] These changes came after 2 landmark randomized controlled trials, DAWN[5] and DEFUSE-3.[6] DEFUSE-3 was stopped early for efficacy when results revealed improved 90-day functional outcomes with thrombectomy 6 to 16 hours after the onset of symptoms. DAWN extended the time window to 24 hours for selected patients. Patients in the positive thrombectomy trials were treated at hospitals with complex, efficient, team-based stroke systems in place.[7] Experts note, to optimize attainment of trial results in actual practice, patients should receive thrombectomy treatment at facilities certified as having the "resources, personnel, organization, and continuous quality improvement processes characteristic of trial centers."[7] In other words, stroke systems of care.

## STROKE SYSTEM OF CARE

The development of acute treatments for stroke has necessitated the rapid identification of stroke symptoms and an organized approach to stroke health care delivery. This has led to a tiered system of certified stroke centers.

As far back as 2000, anticipating the need for a hierarchical organization of stroke care, the Brain Attack Coalition (BAC) provided recommendations for the development of primary stroke centers (PSCs).[8] In the years that followed, BAC published additional recommendations for acute stroke–ready hospitals (ASRHs) and Comprehensive Stroke Centers (CSCs).[8] In 2005, the AHA/ASA brought together a task force on the development of stroke systems.[9] This task force recommended methods for the implementation of stroke systems of care. Nearly 20 years later, the recommendations for regional systems of stroke care remain. The most recent ASA 2018 guidelines recommend that

> "Regional systems of stroke care should be developed. These should consist of the following; (a) Healthcare facilities that provide initial emergency care, including administration of IV alteplase and (b) Centers capable of performing endovascular stroke treatment with comprehensive periprocedural care...."[10]

In 2019, ASA updated its prior system of stroke care guidelines paper to help lead policy makers and health care providers. The update spans primordial and primary prevention, acute stroke recognition, secondary prevention at hospital discharge, and rehabilitation and recovery.[11] The paper notes that given the recent developments in treatment, specifically thrombectomy, getting patients to a qualified provider at the right hospital was critical to the patient accessing the highest level of care for which they are eligible. Furthermore, patients with acute complex stroke, such as those with intracranial hemorrhage (ICH) and subarachnoid hemorrhage (SAH), should be evaluated and treated at hospitals with dedicated neurosurgical and neuroscience intensive care services.[11] Given this, the previously mentioned 3-tier system of hospital certification that has emerged over the past 20 years has undergone further refinement to include an additional certification of thrombectomy capable[11]

The differing levels of stroke certification recognize the variances in hospital resources, staff, and training necessary to provide stroke care. In some states, emergency medical services (EMS) have routing protocols that dictate to what level of stroke center a patient will be taken.[12] If hospitals are not properly certified at the level they are equipped to care for patients with stroke, they risk being bypassed by EMS. Not only does this negatively affect the financial health of the hospital, it can delay critical treatment for the patient. This may be a significant financial and clinical motivation for obtaining certification by health care organizations.

Certification for each level of stroke care can be achieved through independent groups that offer certification programs. Most stroke centers are certified by The Joint

Commission, which has formed a partnership with ASA. The Joint Commission certifies 75% of all CSCs. In addition, Det Norske Veritas and the Healthcare Facilities Accreditation Program offer similar certification programs.[13] In some states, the department of public health also offers certification. Although there are differences between programs, the concepts remain the same across the certifying agencies: each certification program is based on the delivery of consistent, high-quality stroke care based on evidence-based practice. This article focuses primarily on The Joint Commission Stroke Certification in terms of terminology, although the reader is encouraged to review the standards and performance measures for each certifying agency. Whichever certifying agency an organization chooses, it is imperative to have open communication with those who set the standard to ensure the level of quality and attainment make clinical sense for the bedside team.

## LEVELS OF CERTIFICATION
### Primary Stroke Centers

PSCs comprise the largest group of hospitals that are stroke certified[13] PSCs were the first level of care that was created to address the issues associated with poor patient access to life-saving stroke treatment. In addition to the certifying agencies previously discussed, some state department of public health agencies certify PSC hospitals.

PSC certification requires a formalized, programmatic approach to stroke care that can meet the needs of patients with stroke throughout the duration of their hospitalization. As with all levels of certification, the PSC stroke program must use a standardized method of delivering care that is developed from evidence-based clinical practice guidelines (**Box 1**). PSC certification also requires that the hospital has the capability to monitor stroke care through performance measures and provides stroke education to hospital staff, EMS providers, and the community.

### Acute Stroke Ready

Studies have shown that approximately 50% of the US population does not live within 60 minutes of a PSC.[14] ASRHs were developed to fulfill a critical community need within the stroke systems of care. These are frontline providers for many patients and ASRHs must be able to safely administer IV thrombolytics (**Box 2**). ASRHs tend

---

**Box 1**
**Primary stroke center**

- Acute stroke team available 24/7[8,18]

- Access to a neurologist in person or via telemedicine

- Computed tomography (CT) capabilities and laboratory testing 24/7. Availability of CT angiography/magnetic resonance angiography and cardiac imaging

- Ability to provide intravenous thrombolytics

- Stroke unit or designated beds for patients with acute stroke

- Transfer agreement for neurosurgical emergencies/further treatment

- Neurosurgical services within 2 hours

- Annual staff stroke education requirements

- Annual emergency medical services and community education requirements

- Adherence to guidelines and monitoring of performance measures

> **Box 2**
> **Acute stroke–ready hospital**
>
> - Acute stroke team available 24/7[8,18]
> - Access to a neurologist: in person or via telemedicine
> - CT capabilities and laboratory testing 24/7
> - Ability to provide intravenous thrombolytics
> - Transfer agreement with primary stroke center (PSC) or comprehensive stroke center
> - Neurosurgical services within 3 hours (can be by transfer)
> - Adherence to guidelines and monitoring or performance measures[15]

to be smaller facilities with a typical bed count between 30 and 100 and yearly stroke admissions between 25 and 50.[13] They are required to have an acute stroke team available 24/7, a neurologist accessible in person or via telemedicine, computed tomography capabilities to rule out hemorrhage to safely administer IV thrombolytics and have transfer agreements in place with a PSC or CSC to immediately access a higher level of care.

### Thrombectomy-Capable Stroke Centers/Primary Plus

This certification is designed for those hospitals meeting the requirements for primary stroke certification that are also able to provide endovascular procedures and postprocedure care (**Box 3**). This is one of newer certifications that was developed to represent an intermediate level of care between PSCs and CSCs. This certification has been somewhat controversial, as it enables PSCs to provide thrombectomy without meeting all the requirements of a comprehensive stroke center. Evidence suggests that patients treated with thrombectomy at low-volume centers have fewer positive outcomes than those at high-volume centers.[15,16] Since the initial introduction of the Thrombectomy-capable Stroke Centers, certifying bodies have introduced minimal thrombectomy volume requirements to ease the concern that some hospitals may not complete enough thrombectomies to be proficient.[17]

### Comprehensive Stroke Center

CSC certification is the most demanding stroke certification available and is designed for those hospitals that have the ability to receive and treat the most complex stroke patients (**Box 4**). The CSC must demonstrate that it has highly trained staff readily available to care for the patient with acute stroke. In addition, the CSC must have

> **Box 3**
> **Thrombectomy-capable/primary plus**
>
> All the same requirements for PSC plus the following[8,18]:
> - Ability to perform mechanical thrombectomy and intra-arterial procedures and provide post-thrombectomy care
> - Ability to maintain volume requirements for number of cases per year
> - Dedicated neurointensive care beds
> - On-site critical care coverage 24/7
> - Increased staff education requirements
> - Increased number of performance measures

---

**Box 4**
**Comprehensive stroke center select requirements**

- Dedicated neurointensive care unit beds for complex stroke patients 24/7[8,18]

- On-site neurointensivist coverage 24/7

- Comprehensive diagnostic services: CT/CT angiography, MRI/magnetic resonance angiography, laboratory tests, catheter angiography 24/7; other cranial and carotid duplex ultrasound and transesophageal echocardiography/transthoracic echocardiography as indicated

- Ability to meet the needs of multiple patients with complex stroke at one time

- Advanced training for nurses caring for patients with complex stroke

- Participates in patient-centered research

- Neurosurgical services available 24/7

- Treatment capabilities: intravenous thrombolytics, endovascular thrombectomy therapy, microsurgical neurovascular clippings of aneurysms, coiling of aneurysms, carotid stenting, carotid endarterectomy; minimal volume requirements for intravenous and endovascular therapy, clipping and coiling of aneurysms

- Extensive quality improvement program and reporting on 18 performance measures (Joint Commission)

---

the ability to perform advanced diagnostic and treatment techniques, have substantial infrastructure to support the program, and have rigorous educational and patient-centered research programs. The CSC functions as a major resource center for several ASRHs, PSCs, and thrombectomy-capable/primary stroke plus hospitals.

## COST OF CERTIFICATION

Cost of stroke program certification is often cited as a barrier to obtaining stroke program designation. The cost of certification varies among different certifying bodies. The certifying agencies may charge an annual fee and also an additional fee for the on-site visit that often occurs every 2 years.

Range of annual certification fees:

- Acute Stroke–Ready Certification: $3900–$4475
- Primary Stroke Certification: $7050–$8400
- Advanced Thrombectomy-Capable/Primary Stroke Plus: $12,200–$17,550
- Comprehensive Stroke Center Certification: $16,400–$24,700

In reality, it is often much more costly to the organization to build the infrastructure that is required to be successful. To attain certification, programs are required to develop, disseminate, and implement evidence-based policies and procedures. Often additional staff must be hired to administer the stroke program, as well as to meet the demand of the quality standards and performance guidelines. Many hospital administrators, physicians, and nurses ask: Why certify? And does it really matter?

## WHY CERTIFY?

### Certification Provides an Objective Assessment of Clinical Care for Hospital Leadership and Prospective Patients

Health care professionals pride themselves on delivering the best care possible. Intensive care nurses are highly trained, dedicated health care professionals, hence, objective feedback on care is critical to a nurse's professional success and safe practice. A properly run and supported stroke program allows nurses to get real-time feedback on their care plans, treatment, and decision making. Stroke certification provides a strong platform for data-driven improvements in hospital-based acute stroke care.[11]

Stroke center certification requires an organization to report on several stroke performance measures. Many of these measures are nurse driven. The number of measures will depend on the level of certification. PSC certification generally requires the Stroke (STK) measures. CSC certification requires the highest number of performance measures (STK measures and Comprehensive Stroke (CSTK) measures). Those required by The Joint Commission program are shown in **Tables 1** and **2**. Other certifying agencies use similar performance measures.

In addition, every health care organization establishes internal standards and rules for operations. Stroke certification acts as an objective stamp of approval and ensures that the organization meets regulations and standards set by a recognized, external organization.

Certification distinguishes the stroke center from other health care organizations. Critically ill patients and their families want assurance that they are seeking care in a hospital that can be trusted to provide the best care for their illness. Certification can enhance a hospitals reputation by the following:

- Increasing credibility among the referring health care community and with patients.
- Demonstrating the organization's commitment and dedication to providing top-level stroke care.[18]
- Increasing the organization's ability to attract top-level health care professionals.[18]

### Creates a Cohesive, Well-Trained Team

Certification is best accomplished by engaging the entire organization's staff in the journey, including bedside intensive care unit (ICU) nurses who are directly involved in the stroke patient's care.

The physician-dominated model of care has transitioned to team-based care.[19] Literature has consistently shown a relationship between teamwork and patient

**Table 1**
**Joint commission STK measures**

| Measure No. | STK Measure Name | Ischemic Stroke | Hemorrhagic Stroke |
|---|---|---|---|
| STK-1 | Venous thromboembolism prophylaxis | X | X |
| STK-2 | Discharged on antithrombotic therapy | X | |
| STK-3 | Anticoagulation for atrial fibrillation | X | |
| STK-4 | Thrombolytic therapy | X | |
| STK-5 | Timely antithrombotic therapy | X | |
| STK-6 | Discharged on statin medication | X | |
| STK-8 | Stroke education given | X | X |
| STK-10 | Patient assessed for rehabilitation | X | X |

*Abbreviations*: STK, Stroke; X, performance measure applies to the associated diagnosis.
© Joint Commission Resources: Stroke (STK) Core Measure Set. Oakbrook Terrace, IL: Joint Commission on Accreditation of Healthcare Organizations, 2018 from https://www.jointcommission.org/assets/1/6/Stroke.pdf. Reprinted with permission.

**Table 2**
**Joint commission CSTK measures**

| Measure No. | CSTK Measure Name | Ischemic Stroke | Hemorrhagic Stroke |
|---|---|---|---|
| CSTK-1 | National Institutes of Health Stroke Scale performed | X | |
| CSTK-3 | Severity measurement performed for subarachnoid hemorrhage and intracranial hemorrhage (ICH) | | X |
| CSTK-4 | Procoagulant reversal agent initiation for ICH | | X |
| CSTK-5 | Hemorrhagic transformation (rate) | X | |
| CSTK-6 | Nimodipine treatment administration | | X |
| CSTK-8 | Thrombolysis in cerebral infarction posttreatment reperfusion grade | X | |
| CSTK-9 | Arrival time to skin puncture | X | |
| CSTK-10 | Modified Rankin score at 90 d, favorable outcome | X | |
| CSTK-11 | Timeliness to reperfusion: arrival time to TICI 2B or higher | X | |
| CSTK-12 | Timeliness of reperfusion: skin puncture to TICI 2B or higher | X | |

Abbreviations: CSTK, comprehensive stroke center; X, performance measure applies to the associated diagnosis.
© Joint Commission Resources: Specifications Manual for Joint Commission National Quality Measures (v2019A1). Oakbrook Terrace, IL: Joint Commission on Accreditation of Healthcare Organizations, 2019 from https://manual.jointcommission.org/releases/TJC2019A1/Comprehensive Stroke.html. Reprinted with permission.

outcomes, particularly in ICUs.[20] The evidence of improved outcomes sufficiently warrants the implementation of programs that are designed to improve the level of teamwork and collaboration among intensive care providers.[21]

Stroke certification programs highly value interprofessional practice models. The very nature of stroke care requires coordination of multiple clinical services. Collaboration among physicians, nurses, and other health care professionals increases a team awareness of each discipline's unique knowledge and skills and leads to continued improvement in decision making.[22]

Properly formed teams benefit from the knowledge, skills, and experience of a wider range of people to solve their problems. The dynamic interaction of the individuals is often the best way to find effective solutions to problems[19]

A study completed by Kagan and her colleagues[23] that looked at the effect of Joint Commission accreditation on the nursing work environment found that the process created a climate that was "improvement oriented, encouraged teamwork and quality improvement."

### Certification Recognizes Nursing Contributions

The 2019 recommendations for the establishment of stroke systems of care developed by the ASA recognizes nurses as key stakeholders in the process of building regional and state systems of care.[11] At the hospital level, any attempt to obtain stroke certification will not be successful without buy-in and commitment from nursing leadership and the nurses providing direct patient care. Stroke certification programs strongly recognize the contributions of nurses in the care of patients with stroke, and most stroke programs are led by registered nurse stroke coordinators.[24] Advanced practice providers also are highly suggested or required to be a part of the stroke team.[17,24]

Certifying agencies require that each nurse caring for the patient with stroke receive an appropriate orientation to his or her unit and stroke care education. This orientation must be documented.[17] Nurses should have access to stroke protocols and reference materials. Yearly evaluations and ongoing stroke competency assessments also are required.[17]

Eight hours annually of stroke education for ICU nurses caring for patients with complex stroke in a CSC is required or highly preferred, depending on the certifying agency.[24] This can be extremely challenging and an expensive endeavor for the organization. Different teaching modalities can be used to meet this requirement, such as computerized learning, face-to-face or taped lectures, journal articles, review of protocols and guidelines, stroke conferences, National Institutes of Health Stroke Scale training, and Emergency Neurologic Life Support training.

Nurses caring for patients with complex stroke in the ICU of a CSC are expected to be experts in stroke care. Competencies are listed as follows:

---

**Neuro-ICU Nursing Competencies for The Joint Commission (TJC) CSC[17]**

Demonstrate expertise in the following:
- Neurologic and cardiovascular assessment
- Management of ventriculostomy devices
- Management of intracranial pressure
- Nursing care of patients with hemorrhagic stroke (ICH and SAH)
- Nursing care of patients receiving IV and intra-arterial alteplase
- Management of malignant Ischemic Stroke (IS) with craniectomy
- Use of thermoregulation protocols
- Use of IV vasopressor, antihypertensive, and positive inotropic agents
- Intracranial hemodynamic monitoring
- Ventilatory management

---

### Understanding the Key Role of Nurses in Caring for the Patient with Stroke

The nursing plan of care is one of the most heavily scrutinized areas that is reviewed during the certification site visit.

Certifying agency reviewers specifically look at the following:

- Neuroassessment and reassessment
- Dysphagia screening
- Medication monitoring and administration
- Individualized stroke education
- Utilization of appropriate consults: rehabilitation professionals, social work, palliative care, case management, and chaplaincy

### Certification Improves Patient Care and Outcomes

Quality improvement is an important activity for all members of the interdisciplinary team, including nurses.[25] The national project Quality and Safety Education for Nurses, has developed competencies for nurses across the spectrum of nursing education and practice.[26] Sponsored by the Robert Wood Johnson Foundation, the competencies included patient-centered care, teamwork, quality improvement, evidence-based practice, safety, and informatics.[26] Stroke certification programs encompass all of these competencies.

Going through the accreditation process helps to streamline operations, improve the quality of care, and build trust with patients and the community. Certification as a stroke center has been associated with a number of quality improvement initiatives, perhaps most importantly increased access to timely thrombolytic therapy and improved outcomes. The implementation of stroke performance measures used by the ASA and the Get With The Guidelines continuous quality improvement program in addition to the multiple stroke certifying bodies has been associated with large-scale improvement in stroke care.[27] Given the more than 795,000 strokes occurring annually, fostering a system of care that reduces stroke-related deaths by 2% to 3% annually would have a profound impact. It could translate into approximately 20,000 fewer deaths in the United States and possibly 400,000 fewer deaths worldwide.[11]

Stroke certification heavily emphasizes standardized care. The word standards or standardization often has a negative connotation for many people. Some associate standardization of treatment with bureaucracy in health care and believe that it mistakenly means that care cannot be individualized. An appropriate amount of standardization is vital to the foundation of health care improvement and is a primary method of reducing variation in treatment that can cause errors.[28] Developing and implementing a standard set of behavior policies and procedures is critical. Stroke treatment policies need to be consistent and universally applied in order for all patients to receive a high-level care that does not vary based on time of day, unit, or provider.

## OUTCOMES

It has been shown that organized stroke care, in the form of stroke care units, reduces morbidity and mortality associated with stroke. Guidelines from the Society of Neurointerventional Surgery recommend that postoperative thrombectomy care should be performed in a dedicated stroke unit with coordinated interdisciplinary care.[29]

In a study completed in 2016, Chaudhry and colleagues[30] compared the rates of in-hospital adverse events and discharge outcomes in patients with stroke admitted to PSCs compared with those admitted to non-PSC hospitals in the United States.[30] Compared with non-PSC admissions, patients admitted to PSCs are less likely to experience adverse events and more likely to have better discharge outcomes. In another study that looked at outcomes, it was noted that obtaining stroke certification reduces stroke mortality.[31]

An important factor in caring for patients with stroke includes the sequelae of stroke, such as hemorrhagic conversion, hydrocephalus, and malignant intracranial hypertension, which often require a higher level of care in stroke centers prepared to manage these complications.[8] This care requires interdisciplinary decision making best performed by a stroke team that includes expert ICU nurses, neurointensivists, and neurosurgeons[8] Expert nursing care as part of a larger system of stroke care can go a long way in reducing post-stroke disability that would greatly improve the quality of life of patients, and reduce health care costs overall. Certification of stroke centers greatly contributes to this cause.

## SUMMARY

Many academic and community hospitals have obtained stroke center certification. Participation in structured quality improvement programs that also incorporate an objective assessment has been shown to improve outcomes and foster team building.

Although certification programs are not always perfect, they provide a framework to ensure hospitals provide evidence-based stroke care. For the ICU nurse, awareness and participation in the certification programs process is an important part of professional nursing practice.

## DISCLOSURE

The author has nothing to disclose.

## REFERENCES

1. Brainin M, Heiss W. Textbook of stroke medicine. New York: Cambridge University Press; 2019.
2. Hacke W, Kaste M, Bluhmki E, et al. Thrombolysis with alteplase 3 to 4.5 hours after acute ischemic stroke. N Engl J Med 2008;359(13):1317–29.
3. Ma H, Campbell BC, Parsons MW, et al. Thrombolysis guided by perfusion imaging up to 9 hours after onset of stroke. N Engl J Med 2019;380(19):1795–803.
4. Powers WJ, Derdeyn CP, Biller J, et al. 2015 American Heart Association/American Stroke Association focused update of the 2013 guidelines for the early management of patients with acute ischemic stroke regarding endovascular treatment: a guideline for healthcare professionals from the American Heart Association/American Stroke Association. Stroke 2015;46(10):3020–35.
5. Jovin TG, Saver JL, Ribo M, et al. Diffusion-weighted imaging or computerized tomography perfusion assessment with clinical mismatch in the triage of wake up and late presenting strokes undergoing neurointervention with trevo (DAWN) trial methods. Int J Stroke 2017;12(6):641–52.
6. Albers GW, Lansberg MG, Kemp S, et al. A multicenter randomized controlled trial of endovascular therapy following imaging evaluation for ischemic stroke (DEFUSE 3). Int J Stroke 2017;12(8):896–905.
7. Mocco J, Fargen KM, Goyal M, et al. Neurothrombectomy trial results: stroke systems, not just devices, make the difference. Int J Stroke 2015;10(7):990–3.
8. Mokin M, Jacuh E, Linfante I, et al, editors. Acute stroke management in the first 24 hours: a practical guide for clinicians. Oxford (United Kingdom): Oxford University Press; 2018.
9. Schwamm LH, Pancioli A, Acker JE III, et al. Recommendations for the establishment of stroke systems of care: recommendations from the American Stroke Association's task force on the development of stroke systems. Circulation 2005; 111(8):1078–91.
10. Powers WJ, Rabinstein AA, Ackerson T, et al. 2018 Guidelines for the early management of patients with acute ischemic stroke: a guideline for healthcare professionals from the American Heart Association/American Stroke Association. Stroke 2018;49(3):e46–99.
11. Adeoye O, Nyström KV, Yavagal DR, et al. Recommendations for the establishment of stroke systems of care: a 2019 update: a policy statement from the American Stroke Association. Stroke 2019;50(7):e187–210.
12. Hanks N, Wen G, He S, et al. Expansion of US emergency medical service routing for stroke care: 2000–2010. West J Emerg Med 2014;15(4):499.
13. Hickey JV, Livesay SL, editors. The continuum of stroke care: an interprofessional approach to evidence-based care. Philadelphia: Wolters Kluwer; 2016.
14. Alberts MJ, Wechsler LR, Jensen MEL, et al. Formation and function of acute stroke–ready hospitals within a stroke system of care recommendations from the brain attack coalition. Stroke 2013;44(12):3382–93.

15. Jani VB, To CY, Patel A, et al. Effect of annual hospital procedure volume on outcomes after mechanical thrombectomy in acute ischemic stroke patients: an analysis of 13 502 procedures. Neurosurgery 2016;63(CN_suppl_1):149.
16. Adamczyk P, Attenello F, Wen G, et al. Mechanical thrombectomy in acute stroke: utilization variances and impact of procedural volume on inpatient mortality. J Stroke Cerebrovasc Dis 2013;22(8):1263–9.
17. Joint Commission. Comprehensive certification manual for disease-specific care. Oakbrook Terrace (IL): Joint Commission Resources; 2019.
18. The Joint Commission. Stroke certification: achieving excellence beyond accreditation. OakBrook (IL): Joint Commission Resources; 2019.
19. Ogrinc GS. Fundamentals of health care improvement: a guide to improving your patient's care. OakBrook (IL): Joint Commission Resources; 2012.
20. Reader TW, Flin R, Mearns K, et al. Developing a team performance framework for the intensive care unit. Crit Care Med 2009;37(5):1787–93.
21. Wheelan SA, Burchill CN, Tilin F. The link between teamwork and patients' outcomes in intensive care units. Am J Crit Care 2003;12(6):527–34.
22. Hughes R. Patient safety and quality: an evidence-based handbook for nurses, Vol. 3. Rockville (MD): Agency for Healthcare Research and Quality; 2008.
23. Kagan I, Farkash-Fink N, Fish M. Effect of Joint Commission international accreditation on the nursing work environment in a tertiary medical center. J Nurs Care Qual 2016;31(4):E1–8.
24. Stroke care certification programs. Vol. 18-0. Milford, OH: DNV GL Healthcare Inc; 2018. p. 76.
25. Curtis JR, Cook DJ, Wall RJ, et al. Intensive care unit quality improvement: a "how-to" guide for the interdisciplinary team. Crit Care Med 2006;34(1):211–8.
26. Splaine M, Dolansky M, Estrada C, et al, editors. Practice-based learning & improvement: a clinical improvement guide. 3rd edition. OakBrook (IL): Joint Commission Resources; 2012.
27. Gorelick PB. Primary and comprehensive stroke centers: history, value and certification criteria. J Stroke 2013;15(2):78–89.
28. Langley GJ, Moen RD, Nolan KM, et al. The improvement guide: a practical approach to enhancing organizational performance. San Francisco, CA: John Wiley & Sons; 2009.
29. Leslie-Mazwi T, Chen M, Yi J, et al. Post-thrombectomy management of the ELVO patient: guidelines from the Society of NeuroInterventional Surgery. J Neurointerv Surg 2017;9(12):1258–66.
30. Chaudhry SA, Afzal MR, Chaudhry BZ, et al. Rates of adverse events and outcomes among stroke patients admitted to primary stroke centers. J Stroke Cerebrovasc Dis 2016;25(8):1960–5.
31. Man S, Schold JD, Uchino K. Impact of stroke center certification on mortality after ischemic stroke: the Medicare cohort from 2009 to 2013. Stroke 2017;48(9):2527–33.

# Ethical Concerns Caring for the Stroke Patient

Dea Mahanes, DNP, RN, CCNS, FNCS

## KEYWORDS

- Stroke • Ethics • Critical care • Decision making • Prognosis

## KEY POINTS

- Nurses should be familiar with state laws and organizational policies pertaining to assessment of decision-making capacity and identification of surrogate decision makers.
- In shared decision making, clinicians and patients or surrogates collaborate to develop a treatment plan based on medical evidence and patient preferences.
- Skilled communication between clinicians and patients with stroke/surrogates improves shared decision making and may decrease ethical conflict.
- Ethics consultation is recommended as soon as a potential conflict about a value-laden treatment decision is identified.

## INTRODUCTION

The care of critically ill patients with stroke is complex and can present a wide range of ethical issues. Even if consciousness is maintained, the impact of stroke on cognition, communication, or both may affect the patient's ability to participate in the preference-sensitive decisions that are inherent in stroke care. Because stroke is a sudden and unexpected event, family members are often unprepared for their role as surrogate.

The concepts of decision-making capacity, identification of the appropriate surrogate, and informed consent are relevant in the hyperacute phase of stroke management and remain important throughout care. Decisions about treatment, including life-sustaining interventions, must often be made. Prognostication is an area of significant research because accurate prognostication may help guide treatment choices. A shared decision-making approach in which clinicians and families integrate medical information with patient preferences is recommended. Skilled communication, within the health care team as well as between clinicians and patients or surrogates, is necessary to prevent and manage ethical conflict.

Nurses with an understanding of ethical concepts play an important role in the care of patients with stroke and their families. This article highlights some of the key ethical

Neurocritical and Neuro Intermediate Care, University of Virginia Health System, Box 801436, Charlottesville, VA 22908-1436, USA
E-mail address: sdm4e@hscmail.mcc.virginia.edu

Crit Care Nurs Clin N Am 32 (2020) 121–133
https://doi.org/10.1016/j.cnc.2019.11.001

issues in the critical care management of patients with stroke. Because implementation of ethical principles in the clinical setting can be impacted by social and legal context, nurses should become familiar with the laws of their jurisdiction and the policies of their organization.

## CAPACITY, IDENTIFICATION OF A SURROGATE, AND CONSENT
### Decision-Making Capacity

Decision-making capacity is based on the ethical principle of respect for autonomy, which is the right of individuals to make choices based on personal values and beliefs.[1] Adult patients are presumed to have decisional capacity until an evaluation has determined otherwise. State laws and organizational policies define which professionals can evaluate patients for decision-making capacity, but assessment by one or more physicians or psychologists is typically required. In order to be a capable decision maker, the individual must be able to understand relevant information, understand the significance of that information to their own situation, engage in reasoning about the options presented, and make and communicate a choice.[2] Decision-making capacity is context specific; for example, a patient may lack the capacity to make complex treatment decisions but retain the capacity to assign a surrogate decision maker. Capacity may also vary at different time points throughout the hospitalization, necessitating reevaluation. The terms "capacity" and "competence" are often used interchangeably, although "capacity" generally reflects a clinical assessment of the ability to engage in medical decision making, whereas "competence" may also refer to a legal determination with implications that extend beyond health care.[3,4]

Following a severe stroke, changes in consciousness, cognition, and communication may impact decision-making capacity. A patient who is unresponsive clearly lacks decisional capacity, but patients with less pronounced alterations in consciousness or with cognitive deficits require careful assessment to determine the impact on their ability to understand and manipulate information. Severe dysarthria makes it difficult for the patient to ask questions and communicate choices, but this can often be overcome with patience and nonverbal communication strategies. Aphasia impacts the patient's ability to communicate questions and choices, to understand the information presented, or both. The involvement of a speech-language pathologist (SLP) can be helpful when evaluating the capacity of a patient with aphasia because SLPs are experts in determining expressive and receptive language function in both verbal and nonverbal patients. In addition, SLPs can often assist with the development of communication strategies based on the patient's individual deficits and strengths, facilitating accurate assessment of capacity.[5] Consultation with SLP may also be beneficial when assessing patients who cannot speak because of intubation but who retain consciousness. Even patients with locked-in syndrome because of pontine stroke may be able to participate in decision making through the use of alternative communication strategies, although capacity assessments are more difficult in these patients.[6]

### Identification of a Surrogate Decision Maker

For patients who lack decision-making capacity, identification of a surrogate decision maker is an important next step. If a patient has completed an advanced directive (AD), designation of a surrogate decision maker is often included. Depending on state law and the type of document, terms used to describe the surrogate decision maker can include medical power of attorney, durable power of attorney for health care, agent for health care decisions, or proxy. Many ADs also identify a substitute or secondary decision maker if the primary decision maker is unavailable or incapable of fulfilling the role of surrogate. If no surrogate has been designated in advance by the patient, and the patient does not already have a court-appointed guardian, most states have laws in place to identify an appropriate decision-maker.[7] The details vary substantially, but state laws typically include a prioritized list of surrogates starting with the closest family member, often the patient's spouse. Other relatives follow in descending order of relationship. Some states include provisions for assignment of a non–family member as decision maker if no relative is available or willing to serve in that role. Organizational policies often expand on state law for surrogate identification. The types of decisions that a surrogate can make are sometimes limited by the AD, state laws, or organizational policies. In rare cases, no surrogate decision maker can be identified, and the patient is "unbefriended" or "unrepresented," in which case decision making may fall to institutional committees or the courts.[4]

Nurses play an important role in identifying the appropriate surrogate decision maker for patients who lack decision-making capacity. Resources for determining the appropriate surrogate include social workers, risk-management professionals, ethic consultants, and legal departments. Nurses can practice preventive ethics by offering all patients with decisional capacity the opportunity to assign a primary and secondary decision maker by completing an AD.

## Informed Consent

Patients with decisional capacity, or surrogates for incapable patients, have the right to agree to or refuse treatments offered by the health care team through the informed consent process. For informed consent to take place, the individual consenting must have decision-making capacity. Relevant information about the proposed treatment must be provided to, and understood by, the patient or surrogate, and the decision to authorize the proposed treatment must be voluntary (made without coercion).[1] Consent is often recorded through signatures on a document, but informed consent is not a piece of paper; it is the process of communication that occurs between the provider and the patient or surrogate as they evaluate the risks, benefits, and alternatives of a specific treatment.[8]

There are several issues related to stroke treatments that increase the complexity of the informed consent process, including the emotional impact of a sudden, unexpected event and the time-sensitive nature of stroke treatments. In acute ischemic stroke (AIS), the narrow window for reperfusion therapy means that the decision to treat with alteplase (tPA) must be made quickly. Other examples of time-sensitive interventions include mechanical thrombectomy for ischemic stroke and intraventricular drain placement for hydrocephalus related to hemorrhagic stroke. Engaging the patient or surrogate in a meaningful consent process respects autonomy, but must be time efficient to avoid treatment delays. Minimizing time delays supports the ethical principles of beneficence (prompt treatment increases the likelihood of a good outcome) and nonmaleficence (prompt treatment may decrease the risk of complications). The American Academy of Neurology (AAN) issued a policy statement in 2011 indicating that informed consent for treatment with intravenous tPA should be obtained and documented whenever feasible, although a signed written consent form is not required.[9] A recent survey demonstrated significant variability in the informed consent process for tPA administration, both in whether consent is obtained and in the information provided to patients and surrogates.[10] Patient-centered decision aids may be a mechanism to improve the consent process for acute stroke treatment. Decision aids provide a visual representation of the potential risks and benefits of treatment, which may be particularly useful when discussing time-sensitive decisions, such as tPA administration or endovascular thrombectomy.[11,12]

For patients with acute ischemic or hemorrhagic stroke who lack decisional capacity, treatment must sometimes occur before a surrogate can be identified and contacted in order to prevent serious harm or death. In such cases, it is ethically acceptable for clinicians to provide interventions consistent with medical standards under implied consent for emergency treatment.[13] The decision to proceed under implied consent does not obviate the need for ongoing efforts to locate an appropriate surrogate, but allows for treatment to avoid death or significant disability. Requirements for implied consent are often outlined in state law, and most organizations have policies that specifically address the issue of emergency treatment. Specific to thrombolysis for AIS, both the AAN policy[9] and the American Heart Association/American Stroke Association (AHA/ASA) guidelines for management of AIS[14] support tPA administration to patients with disabling stroke who lack decisional capacity when no surrogate is available, provided administration is in accordance with practice standards.

## PROGNOSTICATION

Ethical decision making after a severe stroke depends on an accurate understanding of the patient's condition and potential outcomes, recognizing that prognostic uncertainty is often inevitable. Physicians and other health care providers rely on clinical experience and on evidence (outcomes studies and predictive models) to determine prognosis, but both have limitations. These limitations include clinician bias, clinical nihilism, inadequate outcomes data, limited generalizability of available research, and the fallacy of the self-fulfilling prophecy.[15,16]

Health care providers in the intensive care unit rarely see the full recovery trajectory of critically ill patients with stroke, limiting their ability to predict a full range of possible outcomes based on clinical experience. If the prognosis for recovery is judged by the clinician to be poor, the treatment provided may not be aggressive or a recommendation may be made to limit life-sustaining treatments. If the clinician's judgment is based on incomplete information or an incorrect judgment about the patient's potential for recovery, then the patient's outcome is negatively impacted.[15,16] Time-limited trials of aggressive treatment may support improved prognostication. The Neurocritical Care Society Guidelines for the Management of Devastating Brain Injury (including severe stroke) recommend the use of repeated examinations to improve prognostic accuracy and aggressive management to maintain physiologic stability for 72 hours to allow time for prognostic evaluation, care planning, and consideration of organ donation.[17]

Predictive models are available for AIS,[18] intracerebral hemorrhage (ICH),[19–21] and subarachnoid hemorrhage.[22] However, predictive models have important limitations. Most models are based on outcomes studies conducted in a select number of centers, limiting their generalizability because of potential treatment differences in other settings. Another limitation of predictive models is that as treatments evolve, outcomes should also improve. Prognostic models predict outcomes based on the treatment that was provided at the time of the study, so care must be exercised when applying older models to current patients. In addition, outcome data predict outcomes for populations of patients, but the goal of prognostication in clinical care is to provide information about the probable outcome of an individual.[15,16]

Prognostic models may not reflect the outcomes that are important to patients and their families. Family members of patients with devastating brain injury, including patients with severe ischemic or hemorrhagic stroke, want information about functional outcomes.[23] This information is difficult for clinicians to provide because functional outcomes are more nuanced than mortality data. The broad categories of outcomes reported may not represent outcomes that are meaningful to an individual patient or family.[23,24]

One of the most significant limitations of prognostic models is that they are based on outcome studies that do not reflect the natural course of stroke recovery in the setting of full aggressive care. Patients in whom life-sustaining therapies were withdrawn are typically included. Withdrawal of life-sustaining therapies creates a self-fulfilling prophecy, because almost all patients die following withdrawal of support. With full aggressive support, some of these patients would have survived with varying levels of disability. The impact of limitations of care (either treatment withdrawal or do-not-attempt-resuscitation [DNAR] orders) is highlighted in several studies of patients with ICH[25–29] or AIS.[30] Noting the impact of the self-fulfilling prophecy on prognostic models, the AHA/ASA guidelines for ICH management recommend early aggressive treatment and recommend against new DNAR orders through the end of the second full hospital day.[31]

Reports of the impact of predictive models on the accuracy of prognostication vary. One study of more than 700 neurologists and neurosurgeons showed marked variation in physician prediction of 30-day mortality and in recommendations to limit treatment when presented with case vignettes of patients with ICH.[32] When a prognostic score was included, physicians were more likely to recommend treatment that aligned with predictive models of functional independence at 90 days.[32] However, not all studies demonstrate the benefit of predictive models. In another study of ICH in which physicians and nurses were asked to predict 3-month outcomes within 24 hours of admission, physician judgment was more accurate than 2 commonly used prognostication scores.[33]

A recent review concluded that physician prediction of outcomes, especially poor outcomes, is relatively accurate in patients with devastating brain injury owing to stroke or other neurologic injury.[23] The authors further note that the care team's approach to communication and recommendations for treatment can significantly impact surrogate decision making and thus mortality.[23] Recommendations include transparent communication, providing opportunities for surrogates to share patient values and beliefs, and providing information about prognosis while remaining honest about uncertainty.[23] Predictive models have the potential to improve prognostication, but should be used in combination with other factors such as clinician experience and an understanding of what outcomes are most important to patients and their families.[23,34]

## PREFERENCE-SENSITIVE TREATMENT DECISIONS AFTER STROKE

Aggressive evidence-based treatment of stroke aims to improve outcomes, but may lead to survival with significant disability. As a result, many treatment decisions made after stroke must be based not only on clinical evidence but also on patient and surrogate preferences and values. Examples include intubation, mechanical ventilation, hemicraniectomy, and the placement of tracheostomy and percutaneous endoscopic gastrostomy tubes. Ethical decision making in the setting of preference-sensitive or value-laden decisions relies on effective communication within the care team, and between the care team and patient or family.

### Shared Decision Making

In the shared decision-making model, treatment decisions are made collaboratively by the patient or surrogate and the health care team.[35] The patient and family provide information about the patient's preferences, values, and beliefs while the health care team provides information about the patient's medical condition (including prognostic data when available) and treatment options. A shared decision-making approach allows the development of a treatment plan based on both patient preferences and realistic goals. Although most patients and surrogates want to make decisions collaboratively with the health care team, some prefer a more patient- or surrogate-driven approach, and others prefer clinicians to play a larger role in decision making. Shared decision making is recommended by the American College of Critical Care Medicine and the American Thoracic Society as the preferred approach to making treatment decisions in critical care, although they note that other approaches preferred by the patient or surrogate are ethically acceptable.[35]

### Defining Patient Preferences and Values

Patient perspectives on what constitutes an acceptable quality of life vary. Some patients value life even with severe disability, whereas others might view death as a preferable alternative and thus choose to forego or stop life-sustaining treatment. Decision making is confounded in stroke because the patient is often unable to participate. The health care team and surrogate are left to predict future quality of life within the limitations of prognostication and then to make treatment decisions based on their perception of whether that quality of life will be acceptable to the patient, a process termed affective forecasting.[36]

ADs include a range of documents intended to provide information about a patient's preferences and values if he or she loses decisional capacity. Examples relevant to stroke care include advance medical directives and living wills. Limited information about resuscitation and life-sustaining treatments is also available through state-recognized variations of Physician Orders for Scope of Treatment forms. These documents are useful because they often identify the patient's desired primary and substitute surrogate decision maker, and because they provide insight into what the patient considers important. However, most ADs do not provide specific guidance to care providers and families in making decisions about acute stroke management.[13] Documents often state the patient's wishes in the event of "a terminal condition" or "no chance of meaningful recovery," which can be difficult to determine in the acute phase after stroke. In these cases, the AD can be used as a starting point for discussion about the patient's preferences and values.

In the absence of an AD that provides specific instructions, the surrogate is obligated to use substituted judgment. Substituted judgment requires the surrogate to make decisions based on the patient's values and beliefs, even if the surrogate's own values and beliefs differ. In some cases, the patient has made previous statements about life with dependence or disability. Although helpful in guiding surrogates, care must be used when interpreting these statements. Values and beliefs change over time, especially when one is faced with a choice between death and life with disability. If the patient's values and beliefs are not known, then the surrogate makes decisions they believe to be in the best interest of the patient. Decisions made based on best interests must reflect what a reasonable person would choose in similar circumstances.

### Communication Strategies to Enhance Shared Decision Making

Gaps in communication between the health care team and the patient or family are common and include infrequent communication,[37] poor-quality communication,[38–40] and inconsistencies in the information provided by different members of the team.[39] These gaps in communication have the potential to negatively impact family participation in shared decision making and can cause psychological distress in family members.[41,42] National critical care guidelines for patient- and family-centered care, and for shared decision making, recommend routine interprofessional team and patient/family meetings as a mechanism to improve communication.[35,43] Proactive family meetings held before the need for decision making may prevent ethical dilemmas by improving communication and promoting trust between the care team and the family. An approach to interprofessional team and family meetings is included in **Box 1**.

The nursing role in family meetings has been described by several researchers.[44–46] Nurses often assist with identifying important participants and scheduling the meeting. In addition, nurses can review the structure of the meeting and help family members identify relevant questions ahead of time. During family meetings, the nurse monitors family members' understanding of the information provided and asks clarifying questions as appropriate as well as offering emotional support. After the meeting, the nurse continues to reinforce the information provided and responds to family member questions. Nursing participation in family meetings promotes continuity and understanding of the information provided.

Specific strategies to improve the quality of family meetings include increasing the amount of time that the family speaks while the care team listens,[47] along with providing emotional support and reassurance.[48] To encourage substituted judgment and align decisions with overall goals of care (GOC), it can be helpful to avoid asking what the patient "wants"; instead, ask what the patient would think or say if presented with information about his or her condition and the prognosis for recovery.[49,50] Other strategies to improve communication both during and outside of family conferences include using nonmedical language and recognizing cultural differences.[15,43]

### Decisions to Withdraw or Withhold Life-Sustaining Therapies

Mortality after stroke is often preceded by a decision to withdraw or withhold life-sustaining therapies.[30,51] Both withholding and withdrawing life-sustaining therapies is ethically permissible if consistent with overall GOC. The decision to withdraw or limit life-sustaining therapies can be made at any point during stroke treatment using the previously described shared decision-making process. Consultation with palliative care specialists may be helpful when making decisions about life-sustaining treatment and is supported by 2018 AHA/ASA guidelines for management of AIS.[14] For patients who undergo endotracheal tube (ETT) placement and mechanical ventilation after stroke, this initial decision to proceed with aggressive treatment is often made emergently in the early phase of care. As the patient's prognosis becomes clearer, decisions need to be made about continued respiratory support. Tracheostomy may be pursued if ongoing airway or respiratory support is needed to pursue aggressive treatment with the goal of recovery. If GOC transition to a focus on comfort and allowing a natural death, then withdrawal of life-sustaining treatment, including mechanical ventilation, is appropriate.

When the decision is made to proceed with discontinuation of ventilatory support, both terminal extubation (in which the ETT is removed) and terminal weaning (in which ventilatory support is gradually weaned) are alternatives. Terminal weaning allows for titration of medications for symptom control, but the presence of the ETT may prolong the dying process in neuroscience patients because many are intubated primarily for airway control. An individualized approach is recommended.[52] Medications and other interventions to support comfort are recommended before, during, and after withdrawal of support and should be titrated as needed. Even though some commonly used analgesic and sedative medications may depress respirations, the use of these medications is supported if the intent is to provide patient benefit through symptom control.

---

**Box 1**
**Suggested interprofessional family meeting structure**

*Planning*

- Identify participants.
  - Determine if the patient is able to participate. If unable, identify the surrogate decision maker. Ask the patient and/or surrogate if they would like for additional family members to be present.
  - Identify representatives of the interprofessional team who should be present (at minimum, a provider and bedside registered nurse, with additional team members as appropriate to the setting and circumstances).
- Determine and communicate the time and location of the meeting.
- Arrange coverage for other patient care responsibilities.

*Team premeeting*

- Ensure that all relevant interprofessional team members are represented.
- Establish who will lead the meeting.
- Ensure consensus within the team about the information to be presented and the plan of care.

*During the meeting*

- Ensure that all participants are seated at the level of the patient or surrogate.
- Complete introductions.
- Consider briefly exploring the patient as a person before hospitalization (vocation, activities enjoyed, and so forth), especially if the team is unfamiliar with this information.
- Assess patient/family's current understanding of patient condition and plan of care.
- Clarify misconceptions; provide clinical information.
- Engage in shared decision making if necessary/appropriate. When possible, the initial meeting should be focused on building trust and rapport, not decision making.
  - Ask about the patient's or family's preferred role in decision making.
  - Provide an explanation of the role of the surrogate.
  - Offer reassurance that the care team will provide support and assistance.
  - Discuss realistic options, including potential benefits and burdens.
  - Offer a recommendation with rationale if desired by the patient or surrogate.
  - Provide time for discussion.
- End the meeting.
  - If the conference included decision making, ask the patient or surrogate for their understanding of decisions made or that need to be made. Clarify as needed.
  - Thank the patient/family for meeting and participating in discussions about care.
  - Define a follow-up plan, including the plan for ongoing communication.
  - Provide a mechanism for the patient/family to contact team members.

*Postmeeting follow-up*

- Debrief with other team members to review what went well and opportunities for improvement.
- Complete any follow-up items discussed during the meeting.
- Document the meeting in the patient's chart.

---

Decisions about artificial nutrition and hydration (ANH) deserve special mention because families often perceive ANH differently than withdrawal or withholding of cardiopulmonary support. Food has cultural and social significance for many families and may be viewed as an expression of caring. Religious beliefs may also contribute to concerns about withdrawing or withholding ANH. In these circumstances, surrogates often struggle with decision making. Sometimes these concerns can be lessened by focusing on the overall goals of treatment and by providing other ways for the family to provide physical comfort for their loved one (for example, participation in skin care or oral hygiene). For patients and families who decline ANH, careful oral feeding is appropriate in some circumstances even if the risk of aspiration is high.[34] If the patient's goal is comfort and no escalation of treatment is planned, it is ethically acceptable to support comfort feeding after a discussion of the risks and the development of a plan for managing symptoms if aspiration occurs.

Finally, some patients with stroke are candidates for organ donation either because they progress to death by neurologic criteria or because they are expected to die quickly after terminal extubation (donation after circulatory determination of death, or DCDD). Although a full discussion of organ donation is outside of the scope of this article, it should be noted that mechanical ventilation is continued while the patient is evaluated and the logistics of donation are arranged. Care of the DCDD patient before and during withdrawal of life-sustaining therapy is delivered according to usual standards for palliation of symptoms.

### Conflict Resolution

Proactive, skilled communication lessens the chance of conflict between clinicians and patients or surrogates. However, conflict will still occur because providers, patients, and families are all fallible human beings facing value-laden decisions within the complex environment of critical care. When the potential for conflict is recognized, professionals with expertise in conflict resolution should be engaged as soon as possible. Clinical ethics consultants can often provide valuable assistance in negotiating conflict. Other resources with conflict management expertise and skill in discussing preference-sensitive care options include clinical social workers and palliative care practitioners.

Although shared decision making inclusive of patient preferences is preferred, patients and surrogates sometimes request treatments that the health care team feels are without benefit. Clinicians are not obligated to provide treatments that are medically or ethically inappropriate. In 2015, a collaborative of prominent critical care societies recommended a process for conflict resolution when patients or surrogates

---

**Box 2**
**Nursing strategies to promote ethical decision making**

Become familiar with state laws and organizational policies pertaining to decisional capacity and surrogate decision making.

Support patient involvement in decision making whenever possible, using alternative communication strategies as appropriate.

Offer the opportunity to complete an advanced directive to patients who have decision-making capacity.

Advocate for proactive interprofessional team and family meetings as a mechanism for building rapport and trust.

Encourage family members to talk about the patient and to become involved in bedside care as appropriate.

Involve professionals, such as clinical ethics consultants, as soon as a potential conflict arises.

Participate in ethics education as available.

request treatment that the health care team believes is potentially inappropriate.[53] The process has multiple steps, including expert consultation in an effort to negotiate an agreement, a second medical opinion, review by interdisciplinary committee, an opportunity to transfer to another organization if one can be located, and notification of the right to extramural appeal through the courts.[53] In 2016, the Society of Critical Care Medicine (SCCM) Ethics Committee published a position statement that defines treatments as inappropriate if there is no reasonable expectation that the patient will recover sufficiently to survive outside of the acute care setting, or that the patient's neurologic status will recover sufficiently so that the patient can perceive the benefits of treatment.[54] The limitations of prognostication were noted by the SCCM Ethics Committee.

## SUMMARY

Nurses play an integral role in preventing ethical conflict in the care of patients with stroke, and in addressing ethical issues when they occur. Nurses can use basic strategies to promote ethical decision making in their own practice environment (**Box 2**). Laws pertaining to decisional capacity and identification of a surrogate decision maker vary by jurisdiction, so nurses must be aware of the laws in their practice location as well as the policies of their organization. Shared decision making is the preferred model for preference-sensitive decisions after stroke. Shared decision making relies on accurate information about treatment options and about prognosis from the health care team as well as an understanding of the patient's values, preferences, and beliefs. When ethical conflict occurs, prompt involvement of ethics consultants and other professionals is recommended.

## DISCLOSURE

The author has nothing to disclose.

## REFERENCES

1. Beauchamp TL, Childress JF. Respect for autonomy. In: Beauchamp TL, Childress JF, editors. Principles of biomedical ethics. 7th edition. New York: Oxford University Press; 2013. p. 101–49.
2. Appelbaum PS, Grisso T. Assessing patients' capacities to consent to treatment. N Engl J Med 1988;319:1635–8.
3. Clinical Ethics Consultation Affairs Committee of the American Society for Bioethics and Humanities. Addressing patient-centered issues in health care: a case-based study guide. Chicago: American Society for Bioethics and Humanities; 2017.
4. Boyle RJ. Determining patients' capacity to share in decision-making. In: Fletcher JC, Spencer EM, Lombardo PA, editors. Fletcher's introduction to clinical ethics. 3rd edition. Hagerstown (MD): University Publishing Group; 2005. p. 117–37.
5. Suleman S, Hopper T. Decision-making capacity and aphasia: speech-language pathologists' perspectives. Aphasiology 2016;4:381–95.
6. Maiser S, Kabir A, Sabsevitz D, et al. Locked-in syndrome: case report and discussion of decisional capacity. J Pain Symptom Manage 2016;51:789–93.
7. DeMartino ES, Dudzinski DM, Doyle CK, et al. Who decides when a patient can't? Statutes on alternate decision makers. N Engl J Med 2017;376:1478–82.

8. Hall DE, Prochazka AV, Fink AS. Informed consent for clinical treatment. Can Med Assoc J 2012;184:533–40.
9. American Academy of Neurology. American Academy of Neurology policy on consent issues for the administration of IV tPA. 2011. Available at: http://buyabrain.net/globals/axon/assets/8847.pdf. Accessed June 25, 2019.
10. Mendelson SJ, Courtney DM, Gordon EJ, et al. National practice patterns of obtaining informed consent for stroke thrombolysis. Stroke 2018;49:765–7.
11. Decker C, Chhatriwalla E, Gialde E, et al. Patient-centered decision support in acute ischemic stroke: qualitative study of patients' and providers' perspectives. Circ Cardiovasc Qual Outcomes 2015;8:S109–16.
12. Tokunboh I, Vales Montero M, Zopelaro Almeida MF, et al. Visual aids for patient, family, and physician decision making about endovascular thrombectomy for acute ischemic stroke. Stroke 2018;49:90–7.
13. Wheeler NC, Murali S, Sattin JA. Ethical issues in vascular neurology. Semin Neurol 2018;38:515–21.
14. Powers WJ, Rabinstein AA, Ackerson T, et al. 2018 guidelines for the early management of patients with acute ischemic stroke: a guideline for healthcare professionals from the American Heart Association/American Stroke Association. Stroke 2018;49(3):e46–99.
15. Bernat JL. Ethical aspects of determining and communicating prognosis in critical care. Neurocrit Care 2004;1:107–17.
16. Hemphill JC, White DB. Clinical nihilism in neuroemergencies. Emerg Med Clin North Am 2009;27:27–37.
17. Souter MJ, Blissitt PA, Blosser S, et al. Recommendations for the critical care management of devastating brain injury: prognostication, psychosocial, and ethical management. Neurocrit Care 2015;23:4–13.
18. Fahey M, Crayton E, Wolfe C, et al. Clinical prediction models for mortality and functional outcome following ischemic stroke: a systematic review and meta-analysis. PLoS One 2018;13:e0185402. Available at: https://journals.plos.org/plosone/article?id=10.1371/journal.pone.0185402.
19. Hemphill JC, Bonovich DC, Besmertis L, et al. The ICH score. Stroke 2001;32:891–7.
20. Hemphill JC, Farrant M, Neill TA. Prospective validation of the ICH Score for 12-month functional outcome. Neurol 2009;73:1088–94.
21. Rost NS, Smith EE, Chang Y, et al. Prediction of functional outcome in patients with primary intracerebral hemorrhage: the FUNC score. Stroke 2008;39:2304–9.
22. Witsch J, Frey HP, Patel S, et al. Prognostication of long-term outcomes after subarachnoid hemorrhage: the FRESH score. Ann Neurol 2016;80:46–58.
23. Pratt AK, Chang JJ, Sederstrom NO. A fate worse than death: prognostication of devastating brain injury. Crit Care Med 2019;47:591–8.
24. Knies AK, Hwang DY. Palliative care practice in neurocritical care. Semin Neurol 2016;36:631–41.
25. Becker KJ, Baxter AB, Cohen WA, et al. Withdrawal of support in intracerebral hemorrhage may lead to self-fulfilling prophecies. Neurol 2001;56:766–72.
26. Creutzfeldt CJ, Becker KJ, Weinstein JR, et al. Do-not-attempt-resuscitation orders and prognostic models for intraparenchymal hemorrhage. Crit Care Med 2011;39:158–62.
27. Morgenstern LB, Zahuranec DB, Sánchez BN, et al. Full medical support for intracerebral hemorrhage. Neurol 2015;84:1739–44.
28. Zahuranec DB, Brown DL, Lisabeth LD, et al. Early care limitations independently predict mortality after intracerebral hemorrhage. Neurol 2007;68:1651–7.

29. Zahuranec DB, Morgenstern LB, Sanchez BN, et al. Do-not-resuscitate orders and predictive models after intracerebral hemorrhage. Neurol 2010;75:626–33.

30. Kelly AG, Hoskins KD, Holloway RG. Early stroke mortality, patient preferences, and the withdrawal of care bias. Neurol 2012;79:941–4.

31. Hemphill JC III, Greenberg SM, Anderson CS, et al. Guidelines for the management of spontaneous intracerebral hemorrhage: a guideline for healthcare professionals from the American Heart Association/American Stroke Association. Stroke 2015;46:2032–60.

32. Zahuranec DB, Fagerlin A, Sánchez BN, et al. Variability in physician prognosis and recommendations after intracerebral hemorrhage. Neurol 2016;86:1864–71.

33. Hwang DY, Dell CA, Sparks MJ, et al. Clinician judgment vs formal scales for predicting intracerebral hemorrhage outcomes. Neurol 2016;86:126–33.

34. Holloway RG, Arnold RM, Creutzfeldt CJ, et al. Palliative and end-of-life care in stroke: a statement for healthcare professionals from the American Heart Association/American Stroke Association. Stroke 2014;45:1887–916.

35. Kon AA, Davidson JE, Morrison W, et al. Shared decision-making in intensive care units: an American College of Critical Care Medicine and American Thoracic Society position statement. Crit Care Med 2016;44:188–201.

36. Creutzfeldt CJ, Holloway RG. Treatment decisions after severe stroke: uncertainty and biases. Stroke 2012;43:3405–8.

37. Schwarzkopf D, Behrend S, Skupin H, et al. Family satisfaction in the intensive care unit: a quantitative and qualitative analysis. Intensive Care Med 2013;39:1071–9.

38. Hwang DY, Yagoda D, Perrey HM, et al. Assessment of satisfaction with care among family members of survivors in a neuroscience intensive care unit. J Neurosci Nurs 2014;46:106–16.

39. Hwang DY, Yagoda D, Perrey HM, et al. Consistency of communication among intensive care unit staff as perceived by family members of patients surviving to discharge. J Crit Care 2014;29:134–8.

40. Scheunemann LP, Cunningham TV, Arnold RM, et al. How clinicians discuss critically ill patients' preferences and values with surrogates: an empirical analysis. Crit Care Med 2015;43:757–64.

41. Davidson JE, Jones C, Bienvenu OJ. Family response to critical illness: postintensive care syndrome–family. Crit Care Med 2012;40:618–24.

42. Needham DM, Davidson J, Cohen H, et al. Improving long-term outcomes after discharge from intensive care unit: report from a stakeholders' conference. Crit Care Med 2012;40:502–9.

43. Davidson JE, Aslakson RA, Long AC, et al. Guidelines for family-centered care in the neonatal, pediatric, and adult ICU. Crit Care Med 2017;45:103–28.

44. Ahluwalia SC, Schreibeis-Baum H, Prendergast TJ, et al. Nurses as intermediaries: how critical care nurses perceive their role in family meetings. Am J Crit Care 2016;25:33–8.

45. Krimshtein NS, Luhrs CA, Puntillo KA, et al. Training nurses for interdisciplinary communication with families in the intensive care unit: an intervention. J Palliat Med 2011;14:1325–32.

46. Milic MM, Puntillo K, Turner K, et al. Communicating with patients' families and physicians about prognosis and goals of care. Am J Crit Care 2015;24:e56–64.

47. McDonagh JR, Elliott TB, Engelberg RA, et al. Family satisfaction with family conferences about end-of-life care in the intensive care unit: increased proportion of family speech is associated with increased satisfaction. Crit Care Med 2004;32:1484–8.

48. Stapleton RD, Engelberg RA, Wenrich MD, et al. Clinician statements and family satisfaction with family conferences in the intensive care unit. Crit Care Med 2006; 34:1679–85.
49. McFarlin J, Tulsky JA, Back AL, et al. A talking map for family meetings in the intensive care unit. J Clin Outcomes Manag 2017;24:15–22.
50. Schwarze ML, Campbell TC, Cunningham TV, et al. You can't get what you want: innovation for end-of-life communication in the intensive care unit. Am J Respir Crit Care Med 2016;193:14–6.
51. Alonso A, Ebert AD, Dörr D, et al. End-of life decisions in acute stroke patients: an observational cohort study. BMC Palliat Care 2016;15:38.
52. Paruk F, Kissoon N, Hartog CS, et al. The Durban World Congress Ethics Round Table Conference Report: III. Withdrawing mechanical ventilation—the approach should be individualized. J Crit Care 2014;29:902–7.
53. Bosslet GT, Pope TM, Rubenfeld GD, et al. An official ATS/AACN/ACCP/ESICM/ SCCM policy statement: responding to requests for potentially inappropriate treatments in intensive care units. Am J Respir Crit Care Med 2015;191:1318–30.
54. Kon AA, Shepard EK, Sederstrom NO, et al. Defining futile and potentially inappropriate interventions: a policy statement from the Society of Critical Care Medicine Ethics Committee. Crit Care Med 2016;44:1769–74.

Printed and bound by CPI Group (UK) Ltd, Croydon, CR0 4YY

03/10/2024

01040400-0007